What others are saying.

"Pumps are the gold standard for intensive insulin management and ***Pumping Insulin*** is the definitive user's guide. Walsh and Roberts are to be commended for providing comprehensive, detailed material in a manner so highly readable and user friendly. Beginner or expert, everything you need to know is in this book. Its approach is a welcome relief from traditional technical manuals. With your health care team, ***Pumping Insulin*** can be used as a complete course or as a troubleshooting guide. Careful readers will learn the art as well as the science of pumping insulin from this important book."

> Daniel Einhorn, M.D.
> Director, Sharp HealthCare Diabetes
> Treatment and Research Center
> Assist. Clin. Professor of Medicine, UCSD

"With mastery of the skills taught in this book, my students have been able to accomplish in a few months what I personally had to learn by trial and error over the last 5 years. I rejoice as I see them apply the principles in this book to achieve an improved lifestyle, lower HbA1cs and gain personal control of their diabetes."

> JoAnne Scott, R.N., C.D.E.
> Spokane, Washington

"The authors walk a person through EVERY step in pump therapy with explicit, easy to follow directions. The exercise portion, with practical and precise guidelines for insulin and carbohydrate adjustments, is thorough. ***Pumping Insulin*** is a great guide for active individuals interested in or already on a pump."

> Paula Harper, R.N., C.D.E.
> President, Inter. Diabetic Athletes Assoc.
> Phoenix, Arizona

"Both clinicians and patients can learn about the 'nuts and bolts' of pump therapy by reading this book. I strongly recommend it for any patient considering pump therapy or already wearing a pump."

> Irl B. Hirsch, M.D.
> Medical Director, University of Washington
> Diabetes Care Center

"***Pumping Insulin*** provides a wealth of information for both the person with diabetes and the health professional. A resource that no one involved with pump therapy should be without."

> Chris Sadler, M.A., C.D.E.
> Outpatient Coordinator,
> Sharp HealthCare Diabetes
> Treatment and Research Center

How Will *Pumping Insulin* Help?

PUMPING INSULIN COVERS THESE SKILLS:

- daily monitoring and charting,
- testing and setting basal rates,
- testing and setting Carbohydrate Boluses,
- testing and setting High Blood Sugar Boluses,
- avoiding and correcting low blood sugars,
- compensating for exercise and increased activity, and
- analyzing blood sugar patterns so you can normalize them.

PUMPING INSULIN INCLUDES THESE INNOVATIVE TOOLS:

- the PumpFormance Checklist to check overall control, Chapter 2
- Advanced Workshop Charting for analysis, Chapter 5
- easy carbohydrate counting, Chapter 6
- a novel table that gives starting basals and boluses, Chapter 7
- the 1500 Rule to lower high blood sugars safely, Chapter 11
- the Unused-Insulin Rule to handle overlapping boluses, Chapter 12
- brand new exercise tips, Chapter 14
- how to identify and correct unwanted blood sugar patterns, Chapter 17
- how complications develop and how to stop them, Chapter 20

PUMPING

INSULIN

*EVERYTHING IN A BOOK FOR SUCCESSFUL
USE OF AN INSULIN PUMP*

Completely Revised Second Edition

John Walsh, P.A., C.D.E., and Ruth Roberts, M.A.

With Carbohydrate Counting by Betty Brackenridge, M.S., R.D., C.D.E.

Torrey Pines Press
1030 West Upas Street
San Diego, California 92103-3821
Fax 1-619-497-0900

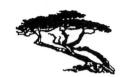

Library of Congress Cataloging in Publication Data

Pumping Insulin
       Everything in a book for successful use of an insulin pump
       John Walsh, P.A., C.D.E. and Ruth Roberts, M.A.

Completely Revised Second Edition, 1994
156 pages
Bibliographical references.
Index.
1. Diabetes
2. Diabetes--Insulin
3. Diabetes--Insulin-dependent diabetes
4. Diabetes--Research
5. Insulin--Therapeutic use
I. Title

CIP 94-60170 1994
ISBN 1-884804-77-2 $19.95 Paperback

Printed in the United States of America

Forward

The insulin pump is widely considered the gold standard for intensive insulin management. There has been rapid growth in the use of the insulin pump as more clinicians and people with diabetes recognize the value of intensive insulin therapy. The Diabetes Control and Complications Trial, summarized in this book, provided conclusive proof that intensive therapy of diabetes prevents complications, and 40% of participants in the Trial used the insulin pump for some time. Virtually all users of the insulin pump feel that it optimizes flexibility and control while minimizing the risk of hypoglycemia. We therefore expect many more people to be pumping insulin in the years to come.

Pumping Insulin is the definitive guide to using an insulin pump. It is written with the intimate understanding and authority of "insiders", authors who have used the pump and trained hundreds of others in its use. It presents technical information in a highly readable manner, and the organization makes it ideal as a troubleshooting guide as well as a complete user's manual. *Pumping Insulin* is comprehensive in scope, but is divided into small, practical sections that take you step by step through the process of using a pump optimally. I expect many sections will be read over and over as you gain increasing sophistication with the nuances of pumping. This should be one of the pleasures of this book.

All diabetes management requires recognition of the art and discipline of caring for oneself, as well as a close ongoing relationship with the diabetes team. The authors fully understand this and weave the understanding throughout the technical details. The book feels very personal, as if John Walsh and Ruth Roberts are actually sitting with you, speaking to you in conversational tones. This may be the only technical manual you'll read just for enjoyment!

Daniel Einhorn, M.D.
Director, Sharp HealthCare Diabetes Treatment
and Research Center
Assistant Clinical Professor of Medicine, UCSD

I have had diabetes for 26 years. The best of those years have been the last three on my pump. The first edition of *Pumping Insulin* introduced me to pumping and was the vital link that put me on the cutting edge of tight control. Now the Diabetes Control and Complications Trial has proven beyond a doubt that tight control prevents complications. This second edition of *Pumping Insulin* provides a whole new world of ideas to reach the best control possible. It takes the guesswork out of using a pump. I highly recommend this book to everyone on insulin, whether pumping or not!

Pat Gallagher
Host, *Living With Diabetes*
CNBC Television/American Medical Television
and EDI Radio Network

Diabetes has affected every part of my life for the last 30 years: my physical health, emotions, family, leisure time activities, performance at work, and outlook on the future. I have used an insulin pump for more than 10 years. I am able to maintain near normal blood sugars and avoid insulin reactions with my pump. I have been able to stop the progression of diabetes complications and improve the quality of my life.

Pumping Insulin tells the reader how to manage their diabetes and how to use an insulin pump. This book is very practical, well organized, and loaded with tools that can be used everyday. The methods described in this book will work for anyone who has the patience and desire to take care of themselves.

An insulin pump is not easier than shots. Taking good care of your diabetes requires more effort than not taking care of yourself. This book tells you:

- how much background insulin you need (basal rate)
- how much insulin to take for food (bolus doses)
- how much insulin to take to lower your blood sugar to normal
- how to adjust your insulin for exercise
- how to handle pump problems like leaks, clogged tubing, and skin irritation

Chapter 20 is worth the price of the book for anyone with diabetes. Besides maintaining near normal blood sugars, there are other things that can be done to prevent, slow or reverse the complications of diabetes. This chapter explains the value of antioxidants, ACE inhibitors, bioflavanoids, antihistamines, and the importance of lowering blood pressure, cholesterol and triglycerides.

The pump and the community of other pump users have been a great blessing in my life. I have been privileged to know the authors of this book for almost ten years. Thank you, John and Ruth!

John Rodosevich
Editor-in-Chief
Insulin Pumpers Newsletter

This second edition of *Pumping Insulin* is more than an instructional manual; it is best viewed as an owner's manual for diabetes. Nothing is considered too insignificant to be included and no area of importance is overlooked. This is what one would expect from two authors who have devoted themselves to helping improve the state of health of people with diabetes.

Pumping Insulin is not meant to be glanced at or filed away. It is meant to serve as a constant resource which should be looked at and evaluated on an ongoing basis. No one person has the answer to all of life's questions; however, as close as humanly possible, this book contains the answers to all of the questions and variabilities which occur in the course of pumping insulin. One can only admire this bible of insulin infusion for its completeness and accuracy.

No machine should come without an owner's manual. This book serves as a learner's manual and also aids the reader to achieve the safe delivery of insulin. *Pumping Insulin* assures the reader a life of good control which as we now know is a life which holds the promise of decreased complications from diabetes.

Alan O. Marcus, M.D., F.A.C.P.
South Orange County Endocrinology

An Important Note

Pumping Insulin has been developed as a guide. Guidelines, examples, situations and sample charts are included to provide basic and advanced information related to the use of an insulin pump. **Insulin requirements and treatment protocols differ significantly from one person to the next.** The information included in this book should only be used as a guide. It is not a substitute for the sound medical advice of your personal physician/health care team. Individual treatment plans, insulin dosages and other aspects of health care for a person with diabetes must be based on individualized treatment protocols under the guidance of your physician/health care team. The information in this book is provided to enhance your diabetes understanding so that you can manage the daily lifestyle challenges you face. It can never be relied upon as a sole source for your personal diabetes regimen.

While every reasonable precaution has been taken in the preparation of this information, the authors and publishers assume no responsibility for errors or omissions, nor for the uses made of the materials contained herein and the decisions based on such use. No warranties are made, expressed, or implied, with regard to the contents of this work or to its applicability to specific individuals. The authors and publishers shall not be liable for direct, indirect, special, incidental, or consequential damages arising out of the use of or inability to use the contents of this book.

About the Authors

John Walsh has worked as a Physician Assistant and Diabetes Clinical Specialist in the Endocrinology Division of the Department of Internal Medicine at a large HMO in San Diego for 10 years. He has used a pump for 11 years, and followed over 150 pumpers and many of the 13,000 HMO members who have diabetes. He has given presentations to physicians, health professionals and private groups including the American Diabetes Association, Juvenile Diabetes Foundation, International Diabetic Athletes Association, and various hospital groups. He is recipient of the 1993 O. Charles Olson Lectureship Award and is a member of the International Diabetic Athletes Association Board of Directors. He has authored or co-authored more than a dozen articles and research papers and two books on pump therapy. He is the author of the bimonthly "Uncomplicating" column in Diabetes Interview. Over the last five years John has been a guest several times on the national radio and TV programs "Living With Diabetes" as an authority on intensive diabetes management. He has provided clinical care identifying those at risk of developing diabetes complications, stabilizing and reversing these complications, and enhancing blood sugar control through innovative methods.

Ruth Roberts is a corporate training administrator, technical and medical writer, and instructional designer in San Diego. She has been involved in diabetes support groups for over ten years and co-authored the *Diabetes Advanced Workbook* and the *Insulin Pump Therapy Handbook*. Ruth is also author of the "PumpFormance" column in Diabetes Interview. She has been a guest on "Living With Diabetes" as an educational expert on intensive self-management. She is a professional member of the American Diabetes Association and past Program Director of the San Diego Chapter of the American Society for Training and Development.

Acknowledgments

Those of us on pumps owe a great debt to companies like MiniMed Technologies and Disetronic Medical Systems who bring us the technology that helps us enjoy better health and freedom of lifestyle. A special thanks goes to Betty Brackenridge, M.S., R.D., C.D.E., of Learning Prescriptions in Phoenix, Arizona, for her excellent work on Chapter 6. Betty is Past President of the American Association of Diabetes Educators, a member of the International Diabetic Athletes Association Board of Directors, and co-author of the excellent survival guide, ***Diabetes 101***.

The authors wish to give their heartfelt thanks to the following individuals who have contributed in their own special ways:

★ to Marilyn James, management systems consultant of Del Mar; Lois Jovanovic-Peterson, M.D., coauthor of ***The Diabetes Self-Care Method*** and Senior Scientist at Sansum Medical Clinic in Santa Barbara; Sally Ann Drucker, Ph.D., North Carolina State University Department of English; JoAnne Scott, R.N., C.D.E. and Jeffrey Hartman, M.D. of Spokane, Washington; Laura Lyons, R.N., C.D.E., Kaiser Diabetes Clinical Services in San Diego; Suzanne Strowig, M.S.N., R.N., C.D.E. of the University of Texas Southwestern Medical Center in Dallas; and Don Leeds of Rancho Palos Verdes, California who graciously and energetically reviewed and improved this edition of ***Pumping Insulin***.

➥ to Linda "Freddi" Fredrickson, Director of Clinical Services and Professional Education at MiniMed Technologies, who deserves special mention for promoting ***Pumping Insulin***. Freddi, on a pump herself, has made editorial contributions to both editions and has pursued making them available to pumpers and health providers alike.

✍ to the American Diabetes Association, the Juvenile Diabetes Foundation, and the National Institutes of Health and other federal agencies that have generously supported diabetes education and research to the benefit of all.

➢ to Reid Wronski, rocket scientist and bridge engineer from Minnesota, who created the Advanced Workshop Chart and shared adventures in pumping and biking with us.

☞ to John Rodosevich for leadership in forming the San Diego Pump Club, and for the wit and humor that has made his *Insulin Pumpers* newsletter so widely read.

➠ to Carlo Luetto of MiniMed Technologies and many other frontline sales representatives at Disetronic Medical Systems, Inc., MiniMed, and other diabetes service industries who care about people with diabetes and show this in the service they provide.

☀ to all the San Diego Pump Club Members and the many other unnamed pumpers and injectors who have made the creation of this book so interesting and enjoyable.

✳ to Irl B. Hirsch, M.D., and Ruth Farkas-Hirsch, M.S., R.N., C.D.E., Univ. of Washington School of Medicine; Davida F. Kruger, R.N., M.S.N., C.D.E., Henry Ford Hospital; and Charlene Freeman, R.N., C.D.E., McFarland Diabetes Center who reviewed and improved the first edition of ***Pumping Insulin***.

✔ to Katharine Alling and the late John R. Williams, Jr., M.D., for helping to birth the concept of an intensive blood sugar control program in the late 1970's.

❤ and especially to Diane Steiner of KD Imagery for her creativity and graphics.

Table Of Contents

Introduction

Pumping Insulin is for:

anyone considering using an insulin pump,
anyone beginning to use a pump,
anyone using a pump who wants to improve their control, and
all health professionals who assist others in using their insulin pumps.

Pumping Insulin gives you a complete system for obtaining the best results from an insulin pump. Read the book first from cover to cover to become familiar with the steps involved in complete control. After understanding these steps, you'll be better prepared to refer to specific chapters within *Pumping Insulin* as you deal with problem areas in your own blood sugar control. Then ask yourself the questions in the PumpFormance Checklist in Chapter 2 for guidance to specific areas in the book that will help you obtain better control.

Our intent is to provide straightforward, useful information. Headings, lists, bullets, charts and graphs are provided for clear understanding of the material. We have chosen nonmedical language whenever possible to assist readers of all backgrounds. You will see reference numbers in several chapters that refer to research articles listed at the end of the book. These research articles are from standard medical journals, and the interested reader may obtain them at any medical school library.

We chose the terms "physician/health care team" and "health providers" through the book to recognize the health care team approach to diabetes care. Although your physician helps you to make most decisions regarding blood sugar control and health care, other members of your health care team implement many of the details of this care. The use of the combined terms covers all the health professionals who assist you.

Before John's patients in San Diego are placed on an insulin pump, they must be willing to pursue using tools and information that take advantage of this advanced technology. To do this, they often attend an Advanced Diabetes Workshop and chart information related to blood sugar control outlined in Chapter 5. This is done for several weeks before beginning pump therapy. *Pumping Insulin* represents the understanding of such an advanced pump user. This understanding provides the most successful results on a pump.

John developed the tools in this book for use by those he helped start on pumps. Due to interest and demand for copies by pumpers over the last 10 years, the book has gradually taken its present shape. The methods presented in this book for improving blood sugars on an insulin pump draw on his 14 years of research, study, and clinical experience in the diabetes health care field. It also draws upon over four decades of personal experience with diabetes. Several hundred pumpers, including many of the pumpers in the Diabetes Control and Complications Trial, have successfully used their insulin pumps by applying the methods contained in *Pumping Insulin*.

Our experience has shown that these methods work well in achieving excellent control on an insulin pump. Progress is being made in other technologies, such as rapid-acting monomeric insulin and non-invasive blood sugar monitoring, that will soon make blood sugar control even easier.

If you have any questions about the importance of normal blood sugars, read Chapter 3 and Chapter 20 first. In these chapters, you will find some of the mechanisms by which poorly-controlled diabetes has its adverse effects. Understanding these mechanisms provides the motivation to keep your blood sugars well-controlled. These chapters also provide additional information in your overall effort to stay healthy.

Read This!

Never use this book on your own! Any suggestion made in this book for improving blood sugar control with an insulin pump should **only be followed with the approval and under the guidance of your personal physician**. We have tried to provide the best information and tools available to make your insulin pump do its job of normalizing your blood sugars. **But this book is not enough.**

We have worked with pumpers who have used this information together with the guidance of their physician and they have excelled. We have also seen pumpers who get themselves into trouble by a selective use of this or other material, and by ignoring or not seeking excellent medical advice. Seek out the advice and guidance of your physician and health care team. No book can ever help you as much as they will. They have the benefits of objectivity and experience gained from working with many other pumpers. Your own participation in the process of good control is essential, but never minimize the importance of good professional advice and support. Teams win where individuals fail, and teamwork takes trust and communication from everyone.

We wish all users of this book good health and great control with their pumps.

Insulin Pump

A small computerized device that delivers Regular insulin via a plastic catheter attached to a metal needle or teflon infusion set inserted into the skin. Doses of insulin, often as small as 0.1 unit, can be delivered with accuracy. Insulin pumps do not measure nor control blood sugars on their own, but must be programmed correctly from information gained through blood sugar monitoring.

PUMPING INSULIN

IS PUMPING FOR YOU?

1

An insulin pump is the best tool available for achieving normal blood sugars. Pumping is preferred to injections because it more closely mimics normal insulin release from the pancreas. Over 18,000 people with Type I and Type II diabetes use insulin pumps in the United States and over 15,000 in the rest of the world. This number has grown rapidly since the results of the Diabetes Control and Complications Trial (DCCT) were reported in 1993. This research showed that people with Type I diabetes had significantly fewer complications when they had control of their diabetes.

When an insulin pump is used well, a person feels better, lives more freely and is likely to have fewer diabetes related health problems as a result of improved blood sugar control. Those who use pumps say things like, "For the first time in years, I can eat when I want to," or "I can really control my blood sugars now, and I feel better too."

People with diabetes choose pumps for:

- a freer lifestyle,
- normal blood sugars,
- flexibility in meal timing and size,
- fewer and less severe insulin reactions,
- the ability to exercise without losing control,
- control while travelling or working variable schedules,
- membership in a community of forward-thinking, health-conscious people, and
- peace of mind.

Health providers recommend pumps to some individuals for:

- preventing, delaying or reversing complications,
- managing the Dawn Phenomenon,
- reducing wide blood sugar fluctuations in "brittle" diabetes,
- tight control during pregnancy,
- improved control during the growth spurts of adolescence, and
- counteracting insulin resistance in Type II diabetes.

Pumps help people with peripheral and autonomic neuropathy,[1,2] early kidney disease (microalbuminuria),[3] and retinopathy.[4] Pumps are beneficial to those who have a Dawn Phenomenon, erratic control[5,6] or insulin resistance.[7] If you are deciding whether to use an insulin pump, you want to consider the advantages it provides in controlling blood sugars and its occasional drawbacks. ***Pumping Insulin*** covers these concerns and provides the tools needed to achieve excellent blood sugar control on a pump.

ADVANTAGES

Many research studies, but especially the Diabetes Control and Complications Trial, have shown how important it is to keep blood sugars as normal as possible. Good control comes from matching the amount of insulin needed with the amount delivered. There are two ways to accomplish this. One is to live a very regulated lifestyle and give set doses of insulin. The other is to live a more varied lifestyle and adjust insulin doses accordingly. Dr. Alan Marcus states this clearly: "A basic tenet of diabetes care is that the degree of lifestyle flexibility that can be achieved is directly related to the number of daily insulin injections." [8]

"Is a pump any better than taking multiple injections?" This is the question most people ask as they consider using a pump. The discussion below details some of the differences between these two methods for optimizing control.

Beta cells in a normal pancreas release **precise** amounts of insulin to cover two needs. First, the pancreas releases a background flow of insulin into the blood when a person is not eating. This **background** insulin directs the release and uptake of glucose and, to some extent, fat as fuels. An insulin pump mimics this background flow of insulin by **basal** insulin delivery.

Then, short bursts or boluses of insulin are released by the normal pancreas into the bloodstream to match **carbohydrate** in food when it is eaten. This larger, quicker release is mimicked by **meal boluses** on a pump.

Obviously, an insulin delivery system must be precise and flexible to meet these needs and match the demands of an active lifestyle. When an insulin pump is used well, **it is the best tool for achieving control and allowing a freer lifestyle**. Let's look at factors that hamper insulin injections in matching insulin need and the reasons a pump better handles these challenges.

RELIABLE INSULIN ABSORPTION

NPH, Lente and Ultralente insulins work over longer periods of time than Regular and are used in injections for this reason. When injected, a **large pool** of one of these insulins is placed under the skin. This pool of insulin is then absorbed from the injection site over the next 24 to 36 hours. Unfortunately, these large pools of insulin result in wide variations in the amount of insulin **actually absorbed into the blood from the injection site**. This is especially true during exercise or when the skin is warmed during hot weather, or in a hot bath or sauna. The amount of insulin that reaches the blood from injection sites **can vary by 25% from one day to the next**.[9]

Because only Regular insulin, which works over 5 to 6 hours, is used in an insulin pump and the insulin pool under the skin is smaller than with injections, there is **less variation in insulin delivery** into the blood. Day to day variation is lowered to about 3% on a pump.[10] Use of a pump avoids more erratic absorption occurring with large pools of NPH, Lente and Ultralente insulins.

MATCHES INSULIN TO NEED

To control blood sugars with diabetes, insulin is used to match **three** needs:

First, insulin covers background insulin requirements. (This insulin lets cells use glucose made by the liver, controls release of free fatty acids by liver and fat cells, balances other hormones found in the blood, transports some amino acids into cells, etc.)

Second, it covers carbohydrates in foods.

Third, it lowers high blood sugars to a normal range.

Meeting these three needs requires precise, flexible insulin delivery. Most people use two to three injections a day for convenience. But then each injection has to cover all three needs. If the blood sugar is high or low, it becomes difficult to determine which need was poorly matched. "My blood sugar's high. I don't know if I covered dinner with too little Regular or if my NPH is too low," is a common dilemma. On a true multiple injection regimen, Regular insulin is taken before each meal along with two injections of a longer-acting insulin. This requires three to five injections a day. Even with great motivation and the use of a Novo-pen® or other multiple injection device, this regimen can be difficult to follow.

Determining the source of an insulin delivery problem is easier on a pump because of the pump's basal/bolus delivery modes. Normally, 40% to 50% of the total insulin need is delivered continually around the clock as **basal insulin**. The speed with which it is delivered is called the **basal rate**. Basal insulin delivery covers the background insulin requirements needed to keep blood sugars level and normal when the wearer is not eating. That's all basal insulin does. It can be tested to make sure it is doing its job by simply not eating.

The remainder of the insulin is delivered by a pump as boluses. **Bolus insulin** is a rapid delivery of insulin, usually before meals. Boluses are used to cover the other two needs:

- covering the carbohydrates in meals, and
- lowering high blood sugars to a normal range.

On a pump, the **basal insulin must first be correctly set** to keep blood sugars normal while fasting. Once the basal rate is successfully set, the grams of carbohydrate in a meal can be measured and matched with a bolus of insulin. The **Carbohydrate or Meal Bolus** works only to balance this carbohydrate. If a meal bolus is incorrectly estimated, blood sugar tests taken 3 to 5 hours later will show an obvious rise or fall beyond an anticipated range. Because the basal rate has been tested and found to keep the blood sugars normal, you know that your bolus for that carbohydrate needs to be adjusted.

If a blood sugar is high, a **High Blood Sugar Bolus** can be taken to bring the blood sugar down based on the number of points (mg/dl) the blood sugar drops per unit of Regular. If no eating occurs, a blood sugar taken 4 to 5 hours after the bolus should be normal.

Because insulin delivery through a pump is steadier and more predictable, the ability to correct high blood sugars becomes more reliable. After covering the carbohydrate and any high blood sugars, the flow of basal insulin from the pump keeps the blood sugar within a normal range in the hours that follow. The precision of the pump in matching these three distinct needs **makes good blood sugar control easier.**

ALLOWS A VARIED LIFESTYLE

Some typical comments from new pumpers go like this: "I don't **have** to eat. I can wait till I'm hungry. It's the first time in years that I've felt hungry." or "It's given me freedom for the first time. I never thought it would make this much difference."

Few people live rigid lives. Work hours vary, meetings and events occur randomly, meals are delayed and missed, and eating is often done on the run. On the weekends people rise early or sleep in late, exercise more or less and at different times of the day. Eating may involve large family meals or late dining after a movie.

Multiple injections allow more flexibility in lifestyle than one or two injections, but a pump is ideal for matching varied schedules. It's easy to eat a meal later than usual because the basal insulin keeps the blood sugars level. If the basal rate is set correctly, a pumper can go all day without eating and still maintain normal blood sugars. Whenever carbohydrate is eaten, a bolus is taken to match that amount of carbohydrate. If a blood sugar is high, insulin measured in fractions of a unit is given to lower the reading without having to prepare an extra injection. Before long periods of exercise, the basal rate can be reduced to prevent a low blood sugar with less carbohydrate having to be eaten. Someone on a pump is neither tied to waking up nor eating at set times of the day, nor to having blood sugars bounce up and down as the demands of an active life are met.

HIGH MORNING BLOOD SUGARS

Some 50% to 70% of Type I diabetics find they need more insulin **in the early morning hours** to offset a rise in the blood sugar.[11] This rise, called the **Dawn Phenomenon**, is caused by an increase in the production of growth hormone and a rise in the production and release of sugar by the liver. If not offset by increased insulin, the blood sugar will rise as daylight approaches. The first blood sugar of the day is usually **the most important one for controlling the entire day's readings.** When high, it can be difficult to bring down. Correcting the high with extra Regular often leads to an insulin reaction in the mid-to-late afternoon. "If I wake up high, my whole day is shot!" is a typical complaint.

Those who have a strong Dawn Phenomenon often find it difficult to match this early morning insulin need with any injected insulin regimen. But with a pump the Dawn Phenomenon generally requires a simple insulin adjustment. Basal or background insulin can be adjusted precisely in tenths of a unit increments. Easy programming allows each pumper to adjust basal rates to meet their own need. A typical adjustment for a person with a Dawn Phenomenon usually involves slightly less basal insulin during the middle of the night and slightly more basal insulin before the Dawn Phenomenon begins. "I can wake up in the morning with a normal blood sugar!" is a common joy for new pumpers.

FREQUENT OR SEVERE INSULIN REACTIONS

Insulin reactions occur when blood insulin levels are excessive. They occur **frequently** if insulin doses are slightly too high through the day. They are **severe** when the relative insulin level is quite high. Reactions happen if too much insulin is taken, if insulin is taken but a meal is missed, if the amount or timing of long-acting insulin is misjudged, or if a pool of insulin under the skin is absorbed quickly, such as when exercise or heat causes the blood flow around the pool to increase. People often admit, "I'm afraid of insulin reactions," as the reason for avoiding tight control of their blood sugars. This in turn leads to an avoidance of blood sugar testing which makes control impossible.

A pump improves the ability to avoid reactions because **it matches dose to need**: basal for background need, and boluses for carbohydrates and high blood sugars. Pumps also enhance the absorption of insulin by giving shorter-acting Regular insulin as tiny droplets for immediate uptake. Small doses of insulin can be accurately delivered. This is ideal for people who are very sensitive to insulin and require minimal doses.

Another benefit noted by those on pumps is that if an insulin reaction does occur, it is usually less severe. As insulin delivery begins to match need, the blood sugar drops more slowly. This gives extra time in which to recognize the symptoms of a low blood sugar. As reaction time lengthens, it's easier to remedy the reaction before it becomes severe.

A person's **awareness of a reaction**, however, may be lowered on a pump. Many pumpers notice that the symptoms warning them of a low blood sugar are **more subtle on a pump** due to a more gradual fall in blood sugars. When a person is first starting on a pump, the risk for insulin reactions is about the same as when attempting tight control with injections. But as experience grows, reactions usually become less frequent and less severe.[12]

DEALING WITH COMPLICATIONS

The presence or beginning of any complication related to diabetes is another reason to consider an insulin pump. All of the complications associated with diabetes---neuropathy, nephropathy and retinopathy---develop in the presence of high blood sugars. Of course, controlling other risk factors is important for slowing or reversing complications. Reduced protein intake, lowering elevated blood pressure, exercise, diet improvements, avoiding smoking and control of cholesterol levels have all shown benefits. But maintaining normal blood sugar levels is the "sine qua non" for preventing complications.

Does a pump help in dealing with complications? Yes, because blood sugar control is central to maintaining health in diabetes. A pump provides better blood sugar control due to more precise control of insulin delivery and due to its convenience in maintaining control while living a normal life. Blood sugar control becomes easier, more systematic and understandable. Having a better handle on blood sugar control increases motivation and inspires those on pumps to use them for a healthier life.

FOR TYPE II?

Insulin pumps have been largely used for Type I diabetes where the pancreas produces little or no insulin. Someone who has Type I is dependent on an outside source of insulin to live, so the benefit of an insulin pump is rather obvious. In contrast, Type II diabetes is more often a result of insulin resistance. Those who have Type II produce their own insulin and may even have higher than normal insulin levels, but the body's ability to use insulin is lessened. Beta cells eventually lose their insulin production due to the stress of overproduction, as well as toxicity from excess glucose. Besides allowing a more flexible lifestyle, insulin pumps have some distinct advantages in those with Type II diabetes who use insulin:

- With the more natural delivery of Regular insulin, blood sugar control is achieved with less insulin, resulting in lower blood insulin levels and greater sensitivity to insulin.
- Weight loss may be enhanced because of the ease in reducing calorie intake, along with less overeating to compensate for excess insulin.
- Less strain is placed on the beta cells that produce insulin. Theoretically, this helps blood sugar control as the years pass because more beta cells continue to function.
- Triglyceride levels, often dangerously high in Type II diabetes, are lower because Regular insulin covers meals better and fasting blood sugars are better controlled.

It should be stressed that the same need to achieve normal blood sugars **applies to all types of diabetes**. The mechanisms for damage are the same, whether a person has Type I or Type II diabetes. Many older people actually have "Type III" diabetes, a milder form of Type I diabetes which develops in thin, older people. They are sensitive to insulin and often benefit from using a device that can deliver the small doses of insulin they require.

DRAWBACKS

Some drawbacks may occur when using an insulin pump. These are:

KETOACIDOSIS

Injecting longer-acting insulins creates a pool of insulin under the skin at the injection site. This pool releases insulin over the next 24 hours for NPH or Lente insulins, and over the next 36 hours for Ultralente. But on a pump, only a small pool of Regular insulin is placed under the skin. **If insulin delivery from a pump stops for any reason, blood sugars can start to rise 90 minutes later.** Three hours after insulin delivery is interrupted, the level of insulin in the blood may drop to only 60% of what it was originally.

As the insulin level drops, cells no longer use glucose as fuel and turn to using fat. As more and more fat burns, excess by-products called ketones begin to rise in the blood. A dangerous acidic state, called ketoacidosis, is created by excess ketones in the bloodstream. In early studies, ketoacidosis requiring an emergency room or hospital visit happened once in every six and a half years of pump use.[13] But pump therapy has undergone major advances which have decreased the risk for ketoacidosis.[14] Even so, ketoacidosis remains more likely on a pump than with injections. Ketones fortunately pass into the urine where they can be detected with ketone test strips. Ketone strips, that are current dated and protected by careful storage in a dry area of the home, should be available at all times and used if ketoacidosis is suspected.

INSULIN REACTIONS

The Diabetes Control and Complications Trial (DCCT) clearly showed that the major drawback in attempting to improve blood sugar control is the increased risk for insulin reactions. This increase occurs whether multiple injections or an insulin pump is being used. Severe insulin reactions, requiring the assistance of another person, were three times more likely in the intensive control group. Severe hypoglycemia occurred 62 times in 100 patient-years, or once every 18 months on average in the intensive group compared to 19 times in the control group.[15] Episodes of coma or seizure occurred 16 times per 100 patient-years in the intensive group compared to 5 times in the control group. Some participants had multiple episodes and many others had none at all. The overall benefits of better long-term health, however, are believed to outweigh the disadvantage of some increased risk of hypoglycemia.

HYPOGLYCEMIA UNAWARENESS

Low blood sugars with little or no warning occur in some people who have diabetes. When a person requires the assistance of someone else to recognize and correct a low blood sugar, the condition is called **hypoglycemia unawareness**. It is more likely to occur in those who have had diabetes for a number of years, or when a meal is skipped for which a bolus was taken, too much insulin is given, alcohol is consumed, or excess activity occurs. This condition carries obvious danger to those who have it and to those around them. Hypoglycemia unawareness may develop more easily on an insulin pump because **fewer symptoms** occur with the more gradual drop in blood sugars.

On the other hand, a pump can also **lessen** the risk for hypoglycemia unawareness.[16] When used well, a pump delivers insulin more dependably and physiologically. This lessens the risk of hypoglycemia and allows the person more time to recognize the symptoms of a reaction. Dr. Irl Hirsch and Ruth Farkas-Hirsch, who follow a very large group of people on insulin pumps in Seattle, feel that "since insulin absorption is more predictable, hypoglycemia unawareness should be considered an important indication for" an insulin pump.[17]

Also, the improved cell metabolism that results from more physiological insulin delivery allows cells to repair, and cell function to improve. A reduction in the frequency of low blood sugars, allows a person to regain awareness of his own reactions.[18] Refer to page 82 and Chapter 20 for information on reversing hypoglycemia unawareness.

If you have ever become unconscious or incoherent due to a low blood sugar and required the assistance of someone else to treat this reaction, discuss this carefully with your physician. You may require someone who specializes in insulin pump therapy to help you manage this more complicated situation.

SKIN INFECTIONS AND ABSCESSES

Skin is a natural defense against infection. When an infusion needle from an insulin pump is placed under the skin, it breaks this protection and offers an open door to bacteria. Skin infections are almost never seen with injections, but this risk increases with the use of an insulin pump. If an infection occurs, an antibiotic may be needed. If the infection progresses to an abscess, the abscess must be lanced and drained. If the infection is severe or does not respond to treatment, hospitalization may be required.

Good sterile technique, covered in Chapter 4, is the most important tool in preventing infections. In the DCCT, a serious skin infection occurred once in every 1,200 years of pump use. But be aware: **infections, rarely seen with injections, can and do happen with pump use**.

SELF IMAGE

Today's beeper-sized pumps weigh only a few ounces and are very portable. Even so, wearing a pump is not always the easiest thing to deal with. A pump always goes with you: on a belt, in a pocket or under your clothes. Some people have difficulty accepting this type of attachment. A small computerized device may be too much to tolerate, especially if a person doesn't wear rings, watches or other jewelry.

A few people are not ready for the social interactions generated by a pump, especially if they feel other people will perceive them as different or as having a "disease." The teen years and early twenties are particularly difficult ages to be different. The perceived stigma of a pump may make its use impractical at these ages. Some people are actively involved in contact or water sports where the presence of an external device can present problems. A pump may seem like an annoyance or nuisance. Most people experience doubts before wearing a pump. Attachment to a pump may seem inconvenient, annoying and potentially embarrassing.

After putting a pump on, however, people are almost always surprised at its comfort and wearability. The feared personal rejection becomes instead the respect of friends and relatives as they notice that advanced technology is being used for blood sugar control. If you have concerns about these issues and many people do, see if your physician/health care team can get you a non-operating loaner pump to try out. Remember: the bottom line is that, for very little inconvenience, wearing a pump will probably improve and prolong the quality of your life.

SUMMARY

Pumps have distinct advantages in the control of blood sugars. Compared to injections, they are more consistent. They come closer to maintaining normal blood sugars. They allow more responsive and precise delivery of insulin. They allow rapid correction of high blood sugars. As blood sugars improve, the chance of developing health problems related to diabetes decreases. Some research studies have shown reversal of diabetes-related complications.

Pumping allows the closest approximation of normal daily life: the ability to skip meals, eat late, and cover variations in carbohydrate intake. Quick adjustments can be made whenever elevated blood sugars, exercise, or unexpected illnesses occur.

Because a pump closely copies the function of the pancreas, it creates freedom for the person wearing it. This may seem like a frivolous reason to someone who does not have diabetes. But to someone who has had to eat meals on a rigid schedule, who must have a carbohydrate snack every night before bed, who occasionally wakes up in a soaking sweat at 3 a.m., who faces high blood sugars every morning, who suffers from lows when exercising, who feels restrained from eating spontaneously, who has returned to consciousness in an emergency room with an intravenous catheter in the arm, or who simply wants to sleep late on the weekend, **wearing a pump is a pleasure!**

Pumps have drawbacks. The risk of ketoacidosis is increased, as well as the incidence of skin infections. Constantly having to wear an external device can be a drawback to some. These risks can be prevented or managed through motivation and training. When all the advantages and drawbacks are carefully weighed, **a pump clearly offers advantages in the quest for a healthy lifestyle with normal blood sugars**.

"An optimist is a fellow who believes a housefly is looking for a way out."

George Jean Nathan

PUMPING INSULIN

THE PUMPFORMANCE CHECKLIST:
GETTING FULL USE OF YOUR PUMP

2

Because an insulin pump is the most technologically advanced approach to blood sugar control, proper use requires expertise in setting it up, testing the results, problem solving and using trial and error. Fine tuning of the pump for ongoing changes in daily lifestyle is also needed. A primary concern for all pumpers is, "How do I get the most out of my pump? Since I am investing time and money in this technology, how can I be sure I'm getting maximum blood sugar control?"

To address this concern, we've developed the **PumpFormance Checklist**. The Checklist sets goals for optimum pump use. If you're beginning to use a pump, look at the Checklist to see the level of control you are working toward. If already on a pump, ask yourself these questions to assess your level of control and to pinpoint areas for improvement. If you're a physician or health provider, these questions help in setting realistic goals with the pump users you assist.

Questions in the Checklist are presented in sequential order. Each should be answered "Yes," before going to the next. If you encounter a "No," correct your control at that step before proceeding. For example, if your basal rates are incorrectly set, it won't be possible to correctly set your boluses until the basal rates are correct. Each "No" directs you to the sections in the book to review to improve your blood sugar control.

The PumpFormance Checklist

1: Night Basal

Can you go to bed with a blood sugar of 80 to 120, eat little or no snack and wake up in the morning with a normal reading? —— **No** ——▶ Review Chapters 7 & 8

Yes ↓

2: Day Basal

With a normal blood sugar before a meal, can you skip that meal (no meal bolus, of course), and have your blood sugar stay level or fall no more than 30 points over the next 4 to 5 hours? —— **No** ——▶ Review Chapters 7 & 8

Yes ↓

3: Carbohydrate Counting

Can you determine the grams of carbohydrate in foods you are eating, either through carb counting, food exchanges or by using another dietary system? —— **No** ——▶ Review Chapter 6

Yes ↓

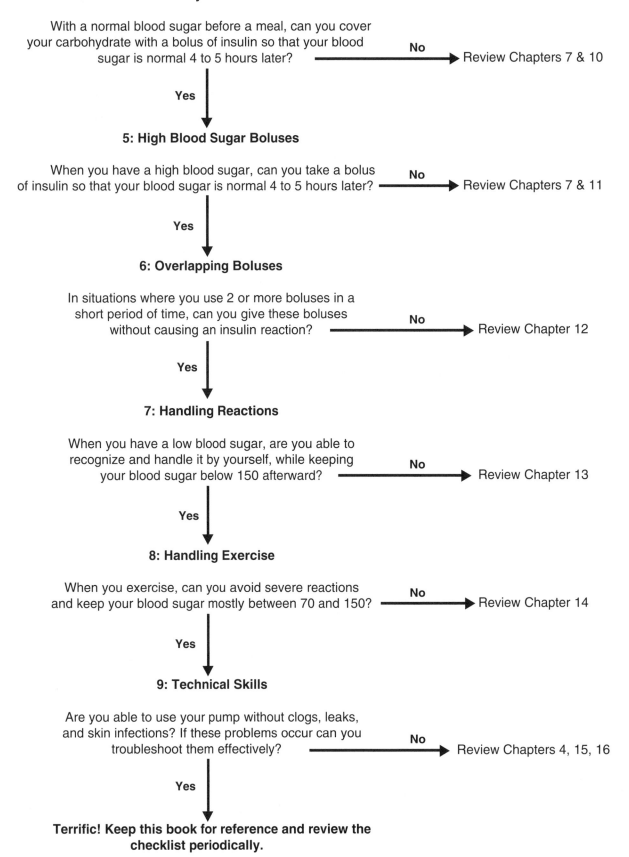

4: Carbohydrate Boluses

With a normal blood sugar before a meal, can you cover your carbohydrate with a bolus of insulin so that your blood sugar is normal 4 to 5 hours later? —— **No** → Review Chapters 7 & 10

Yes ↓

5: High Blood Sugar Boluses

When you have a high blood sugar, can you take a bolus of insulin so that your blood sugar is normal 4 to 5 hours later? —— **No** → Review Chapters 7 & 11

Yes ↓

6: Overlapping Boluses

In situations where you use 2 or more boluses in a short period of time, can you give these boluses without causing an insulin reaction? —— **No** → Review Chapter 12

Yes ↓

7: Handling Reactions

When you have a low blood sugar, are you able to recognize and handle it by yourself, while keeping your blood sugar below 150 afterward? —— **No** → Review Chapter 13

Yes ↓

8: Handling Exercise

When you exercise, can you avoid severe reactions and keep your blood sugar mostly between 70 and 150? —— **No** → Review Chapter 14

Yes ↓

9: Technical Skills

Are you able to use your pump without clogs, leaks, and skin infections? If these problems occur can you troubleshoot them effectively? —— **No** → Review Chapters 4, 15, 16

Yes ↓

Terrific! Keep this book for reference and review the checklist periodically.

PUMPING INSULIN

WHY NORMAL BLOOD SUGARS?

3

Normal blood sugar levels are amazingly stable, staying between 65 mg/dl and 100 mg/dl before meals and rarely rising above 140 mg/dl after even the heaviest meal. These stable levels reflect a precise system that allows the human body to constantly and reliably supply fuel to cells. Figure 3.1 shows this precise blood sugar control.

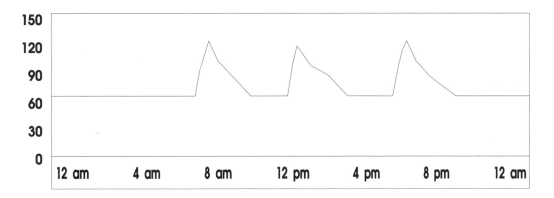

Figure 3.1 Normal Blood Sugar Pattern (with 3 meals)

For a person with diabetes, keeping blood sugars near normal can be a challenge. To handle the challenge, it helps to know how important normal blood sugars are to your health and wellbeing. This chapter presents a few of the reasons why it's worthwhile to spend the time and energy keeping blood sugars normal. In this chapter, we'll discuss:

- how fuel enters the cell,
- how high blood sugars cause harm,
- results from the Diabetes Control and Complications Trial and
    other research studies, and
- a discussion of whether damage can be stopped or reversed.

FUEL AND THE CELL

The health of cells depends on a steady fuel supply from both glucose and free fatty acids. A major regulator of both fuels is insulin released from beta cells in the pancreas directly into the blood. From the bloodstream, insulin molecules cross blood vessel walls and attach to insulin receptors on the outer walls of muscle, liver and fat cells. These receptors then trigger the movement of glucose inside these cells, where it is converted into the energy needed for metabolism, repairs and defense.

11

In contrast to a complicated transport system for glucose, and to the chagrin of many, fat moves easily across cell membranes. Low insulin levels cause less glucose to enter cells, increase production of glucose by the liver, and indirectly increase release of fat from fat cells.

Cells like those in muscle, liver and fat require insulin to receive glucose. (Yes, fat cells need glucose, too.) Other cells such as those in the brain, nervous system, heart, blood vessels and kidneys, however, pick up glucose directly from the blood **without using insulin**.

The cells that don't need insulin to move glucose across their outer membrane **are more likely to be damaged by high blood sugars.** Whenever blood sugars are high, these cells are exposed to high internal levels of glucose. This is one reason damage occurs to nerves, kidneys and to blood vessels in the eyes in poorly controlled diabetes. Cells that need insulin (muscle, liver, and fat) are not as exposed to high internal glucose levels because when blood sugars are high, insulin levels are low. This slows the movement of glucose into these cells.

Cells in the brain and nervous system are also distinct in that they use **only glucose** for energy. (The heart primarily uses free fatty acids.) Hence, the immediate negative effect on consciousness and reasoning when blood sugars are low. As precise fuel delivery is lost in diabetes, blood sugars rise to levels higher than those suited for long-term survival. Unhealthy changes begin to occur. Major physical damage can happen over a few years' time when blood sugar control is poor. Let's look at how complications are related to blood sugar control.

WHAT's KNOWN:

HIGH BLOOD SUGARS HARM YOU.

Hundreds of research studies have shown that diabetic complications occur only in the presence of high blood sugars. The recent findings of the Diabetes Control and Complications Trial (DCCT) as well as many other studies have proven beyond a doubt the health benefits obtained from good control.

THE DCCT

Controlling blood sugars lessens the risk for complications. That's not really news, but the exciting finding of the DCCT was **how much complications were reduced** when blood sugars were controlled. Results of the $167 million DCCT were reported at the annual American Diabetes Association meeting in June, 1993.[15] The study was designed to test whether the effort spent keeping blood sugars normal pays off by limiting health damage. A group of 1,441 people with Type I diabetes were followed for 3 to 9 years. Half were randomly assigned to a "control" group in which blood sugars were moderately controlled on one or two injections a day. The other half were assigned to an intensive control group with the task of keeping their blood sugars as normal as possible using multiple injections or insulin pumps. They were provided the assistance, information and tools to accomplish this task. In the intensive control group, 34% chose to use an insulin pump for control through the entire study.

Compared to the moderate control group, the intensive control group had **76% less retinopathy, 54% less kidney disease and 60% less neuropathy**.[15] This confirms what other studies have shown: complications involving the eyes,[6,19,20,21] kidneys,[22,23,24] and nerves[25,26] occur **only** in the presence of high blood sugars, suggesting that this is the **most important trigger** for these characteristic complications of diabetes. Data collected on eye disease and kidney disease in the DCCT **show a clear linear relationship between the level of blood sugar control and the extent of eye damage and kidney disease**. In other words, for each rise in the average blood sugar level, eye and kidney damage become both more likely and more severe. (The same is believed to be true for nerve damage, but its exact relationship to blood sugar control could not be determined in the DCCT because of the way in which neuropathy was measured.)

Heart disease has a more complicated relationship with blood sugar control because of the many pathways involved. Heart disease can happen to anyone, but heart attacks and strokes occur earlier, more often and with greater severity in those with diabetes. The causes for the accelerated risk in diabetes are complex, and therefore harder to relate directly to blood sugar control. In the DCCT, 14 heart attacks occurred in the moderate control group and only 3 in the intensive control group. This suggests that better blood sugars protect against heart attacks. But results did not reach statistical significance before the study was ended, due to the small numbers of heart attacks in this relatively young population with an average age of 27.

The reduced risk for complications in the intensive control group is especially surprising, given that their average blood sugar (before and after meals) was 156 mg/dl, some 40% higher than the upper limits for normal. Although 40% of the intensive group had a normal average blood sugar range at some time during the study, only 5% were able to keep their blood sugar normal during the entire study. Another 15% achieved relatively good control. **With better blood sugars, results would have been astounding!** The DCCT gives emphatic proof to the decades of observations that people with diabetes who keep their blood sugars close to normal do not develop complications. And though the DCCT study was completed with people having Type I diabetes, most diabetes specialists believe the results **apply directly to Type II diabetes as well**.

An interesting sidelight to the DCCT was the minimal impact that improving technology made during the course of the study in the moderate control group. "Traditional" therapy was used in this group. At the start of the DCCT, this meant urine testing and one or two injections a day. By the end of the study, however, 83% of the moderate group were doing blood sugar testing and 91% were on two shots a day. **But this improved technology had no effect on their blood sugar control!** Although other research has clearly shown that frequent monitoring benefits blood sugar control,[27] the mere testing of blood sugars in the DCCT study had little or no effect on control. It takes specific training in blood sugar control, a strong internal motivation, or the help of well-trained health professionals to accomplish this. The lesson appears to be: **Visit your specialized diabetes clinic regularly to get better blood sugars and fewer complications**.

OTHER RESEARCH

Many other research studies have also linked high blood sugars and damage. One study that matched the risk of developing complications to specific blood sugar levels was the work done by epidemiologists Drs. Hans Janka, James Warram, Lawrence Rand, and Andrew Krolewski at the Joslin Diabetes Center in Boston. In a report in the April, 1989, issue of *Diabetes*, these researchers related the risk of developing severe eye disease to the blood sugar levels of 153 people who had had Type I diabetes for 16 to 60 years.

They divided this group into 4 smaller groups according to how well their average

HbA1c Level in Joslin Study	Ratio of HbA1c to The Upper Limit of A Nomal Range*	Risk of Severe Eye Damage
6.2-8.3	.84-1.12	1.0
8.4-9.0	1.13-1.22	5.3
9.1-9.8	1.23-1.33	16.4
9.9-13.6	1.34-1.84	26.1

Table 3.1 Joslin Diabetes Center: Risk for eye damage in relation to HbA1c level (Joslin nl = 5.4-7.4) Adapted from Janka et al. (ref 28).

* This column can be used to compare your HbA1c level to the upper limit for normal at your own lab.

blood sugar level was controlled, as measured by the HbA1c, during the study period. They followed each group over the next 4 years and monitored which group had eye changes that worsened to a severe stage of damage. The group with the lowest HbA1c levels was given a relative risk for eye damage of 1.0. The risk for the other 3 groups in developing eye damage was then determined. Table 3.1 shows the risk of these groups relative to the lowest HbA1c group.

The speed with which the risk of eye damage increased as the HbA1c rose above the normal range (normal = 5.4 to 7.4% in this study) was surprising to these researchers. A person with a HbA1c of 8.4% to 9.0% had 5 times the risk for eye damage as someone in the 6.2% to 8.3% range. Dr. Warram believes that the risk of eye damage can be quickly reduced by dropping the average blood sugar level. For instance, if the HbA1c is lowered from 10.5% to 9.5%, a substantial drop is likely to occur in the risk of serious eye damage.

A 1986 study by Finnish researchers compared 44 Type I patients with severe eye disease to 45 others who had none. The two groups were identical in how long they had had diabetes, the age at which they developed it, their weight, and the number of men to women. But one thing was different: the group with severe eye damage had **higher average blood sugars**. The HbA1c values averaged 11.6% in the group with severe eye damage and 10.0% in the group without eye damage over the 5 years of study. The higher HbA1c group also had more loss of kidney function (50% vs. 10%), more neuropathy (74% vs. 37%), more limited joint mobility (44% vs. 4%), and higher cholesterol levels.[29] The researchers looked at genetic patterns in each group to see if any association exists between the risk for complications and inherited genes. They found none.

A study reported in 1988 from Dusseldorf, Germany, looked at the way changes in blood sugar control affects eye damage.[30] They followed 32 people with Type I diabetes who chose to go on insulin pumps. These pumpers were followed for an average of 4 years with eye exams at yearly intervals. Any deterioration in either eye was noted, and at the end of the study their eye changes were related to **their average HbA1c levels in the year before their eye damage worsened**. Table 3.2 gives the results.

A marked increase in the risk for eye damage occurred in those who were in poor control **in the previous 12 months**, suggesting that complications depend on recent blood sugar control. Genetic markers were also checked in this study, but again no association with eye damage was found.

Another work focusing on eye damage was the massive study of Dr. Jean Pirart in France. Dr. Pirart followed 4,400 of his patients between 1947 and 1973. He found that factors like age, sex and obesity **played no role in the development of complications**. But poor blood sugar control over the years was strongly associated with eye and nerve damage. Interestingly, the previous year's blood sugar control was again strongly linked to complications in this study.[31]

Risk of Eye Damage Worsening In Relation to Blood Sugar Control in the Last Year	
HbA1c in the last year (normal = 4.2-5.6%)	% of people whose eyes got worse
< 6.13	9.5%
6.13 - 7.35	18.6%
> 7.35	33%

Table 3.2 How Blood Sugar Control In The Last Year Affects Risk For Eye Damage. Adapted from Chantelau et al (ref 30)

Other research also suggests that the damage found in diabetes results largely from an environment of high blood sugars rather than from inherited genes. People who have high blood sugars due to pancreatitis or other injuries to the pancreas **develop the same complications found in diabetes, despite having none of the genetic risks**.[32]

How important high blood sugars are to the development of complications is emphasized in studies of transplanted kidneys. When a kidney is taken from someone without diabetes and transplanted into someone with diabetes, kidney damage typical in diabetes begins to develop in this non-diabetic kidney.

Just the opposite occurs when a kidney is transplanted in the other direction. A kidney is rarely taken from a diabetic donor to give to a nondiabetic. But this was done in Saudi Arabia where a kidney from a young diabetic who died in an accident was transplanted into a person who did not have diabetes. At the time of transplant, the donated kidney showed abnormal changes due to diabetic kidney disease. But when the kidney was again biopsied after several months in the non-diabetic's body, **there was no sign of damage due to diabetes**.

Further support for this comes from the University of Minnesota Hospital in Minneapolis. Drs. Rudolf Bilous, Michael Mauer and others have been doing combined kidney and pancreas transplants for over a decade. People who have advanced kidney disease from diabetes are also likely to develop kidney damage in the donated kidney. With only a kidney transplant, typical diabetes damage is seen in biopsies done only months after the transplant. But when a group of 12 people with diabetes who received **both a kidney and a pancreas** were compared with 13 others who received **only a kidney transplant**, a major difference was found. Compared to those getting only the kidney, **those who received both organs and had normal blood sugars were found to have no damage to their kidneys for periods as long as 10 years**.

These studies suggest that kidney damage is not dependent on the genes in the donated kidney. The major influence appears to be the **environment of normal or abnormal blood sugars into which the kidney is placed**. The Saudi Arabia study implies something else very exciting: that some damage may be reversible.

BUT IS IT ONLY HIGH BLOOD SUGARS?

Although most people with diabetes who have high blood sugars over several years show damage, the damage does not always hit the same organs nor is it always serious. Some people escape serious health problems despite poor blood sugar control. Others will have only a single serious complication. Still others develop all the complications typical of diabetes, involving the eyes, kidneys, nerves and blood vessels.

High blood sugars have to be present to start damage, **but other factors influence the risk for complications**. High blood sugars place a major stress on the body. Strengths or weaknesses within a person's cells determine the location and extent of the damage. The controls over these internal strengths and weaknesses are beginning to be understood. When diabetes is poorly controlled, these other factors begin playing a larger role in causing or preventing damage. Identified factors that determine risk include diet, exercise, blood pressure, smoking, alcohol intake, hormone levels, vitamin and mineral balance, stress levels and genetics. Note that most of these secondary risk factors for complications **can be controlled**. See Chapter 20 for more information on this.

CAN EXISTING DAMAGE BE STOPPED OR REVERSED?

Obviously there are limits to reversing damage. Cells like those in the eye and kidney can't be replaced or repaired when damage has become severe. After a cell in the eye has been destroyed, vision cannot be restored to that area. But can damage to surrounding eye cells be stopped? And if an eye cell is only partially damaged, can it be repaired? The remarkable ability of the human body to repair itself suggests that this could occur.

A research study done in Oslo, Norway in 1984 and 1985 looked at this possibility. Here, 45 people with Type I diabetes were randomly assigned to a conventional therapy group of 2 shots a day or to an intensive therapy group using an insulin pump or taking 5 to 6 injections a day.

When nerve function was tested, the pump users showed **no deterioration at 1 year, a slight improvement at 2 years, and continued nerve improvement over 3 and 4 years of improved control.**[12] **Improved kidney function** was noted after 4 years in the group that used insulin pumps.[33] Their eyes were checked at the beginning of the study and at yearly intervals over the next 4 years. After 4 years, the intensive treatment group had additional minor eye damage but **less** damage than the conventional treatment group. Other studies have also found less eye damage in pump patients with good control.[21] In an Italian study of people on pumps, nerve damage improved rapidly with better blood sugar control and then continued to improve over the remaining 6 months of study.[34]

Research on kidney disease has also been promising. Kidney disease is the most devastating complication of diabetes. Measurable kidney damage is found in 43% of Type I diabetics who have had their disease longer than 5 years[35] and in 25% of those with Type II diabetes for 12 years.[36] **Diabetes is the most common cause of kidney failure in the United States.** Kidney damage goes through stages that can be monitored with standard lab tests:

1. **Microalbuminuria:** Trace amounts of a protein called albumin begin leaking through the damaged filtering structures of the kidneys. Screening for early kidney damage is done with a random urine test for microalbumin (normal on this test is less than 15-30 mg/l). **This microalbumin test is very important and is normally done each year in those who have had diabetes longer than 5 years.** If kidney damage progresses, as it commonly does when intervention is not started, microalbumin spillage will rise above 200 mg/l and be followed by:

2. **Proteinuria:** The spillage of larger quantities of protein is picked up on a standard urinalysis (normal = less than 100-150 mg/day, depending on the lab). As damage progresses and protein spillage reaches levels of about 2000-4000 mg/day, proteinuria is followed by:

3. **A rising blood creatinine:** Creatinine is a normal breakdown product from muscle which the kidneys cleanse from blood (a normal creatinine = 1.1-1.3 mg/dl or less, depending on the lab). As the kidneys have more trouble cleansing the blood, creatinine levels rise. In time, when the buildup of a variety of toxins in the blood become severe (usually at a creatinine level between 3 and 8), this is followed by:

4. **Dialysis or a kidney transplant:** These technologies replace the severely damaged kidneys in cleansing the blood. They also, unfortunately, involve major lifestyle disruptions and cost $25,000 to $45,000 each year.

One of the book's authors (JW) was interested in trying to slow or reverse kidney damage at Kaiser's Department of Internal Medicine in San Diego. With the help of Dr. R. J. Dudl, a pilot study was undertaken. Interventions to reverse kidney damage were started in a group of 16 people with proteinuria (the second stage above). At the start of the study, 24-hour urine proteins in the group ranged from 336 to 3,914 mg/day (normal = 50-100 mg/day). There were 8 men and 8 women in the study; 7 had Type I diabetes and 9 had Type II. The average age was 53 years (range: 24 to 73 years) and average duration of diabetes was 17 years (range: 6 to 29 years).

Normally, when protein is in the urine due to diabetic kidney disease, the kidney disease has an unremitting course unless treated. There is an average of 5 to 10 years between spilling 500 mg of protein per day and kidney failure in untreated Type I diabetes.[37] Diets low in protein, however, and lower blood pressure each slow kidney damage. Diet changes involve a largely "vegetarian" diet with about 4 ounces of animal products from meat, cheese, or milk (1 cup = 1 ounce) per day.

Blood pressure treatment alone is estimated to delay dialysis by one year for every year of treatment. Most of the people in this study (11 of 16) received an angiotensin converting enzyme inhibitor or ACE inhibitor. ACE inhibitors have been especially promising in protecting the kidneys. Blood sugars were improved with insulin adjustments, diet and exercise. During a follow-up period of 5 to 16 months, the change in each person's 24-hour urine protein was monitored and is shown in Figure 3.2.

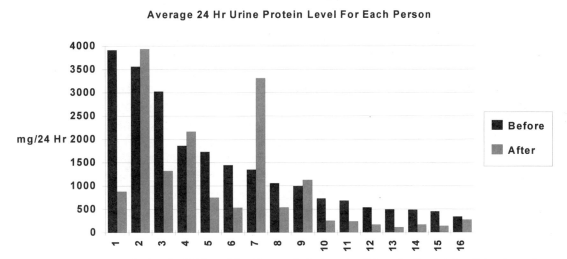

Average 24 Hr Urine Protein Level For Each Person

Figure 3.2 Urine protein levels (24-hour) in 16 people before (solid) and after (striped) treatment. Lower values are better. (Normal 24-hour protein values in this study: 50 to 100 mg.)

When caused by kidney disease and untreated, excess protein spilling into the urine usually doubles each year. After a multiple treatment protocol in these 16 people, however, less protein was found in all but four (numbers 2, 4, 7 and 9 in Figure 1). The pilot study showed a marked rise of 145% in proteinuria in one person (#7), a mild rise of 12% in 3 people (numbers 2, 4, & 9), but **a marked drop in proteinuria of 61% in the remaining 12 people**. The Norway study noted earlier showed similar improvements in renal function in patients in the earlier stage of microalbuminuria, just by improving their blood sugar control. Another study done in Italy in the late 1970's also showed early kidney disease could be reversed with good blood sugar control.[38]

To stop or reverse complications, research studies face a major challenge in the attempt to control blood sugars. Normal blood sugars **are not achieved** by most intensively treated subjects in studies like those done in Oslo, Norway, or by the DCCT. And despite the best of interventions, blood sugars averaging near the normal HbA1c range will often swing above and below true normal blood sugars. "Great mean, lousy standard deviation," as the statisticians say. When these two problem areas of higher than normal average blood sugars and widely swinging readings are improved, further health benefits are likely. ***Pumping Insulin*** is designed to provide the tools needed to improve blood sugar control while reducing blood sugar swings.

Common sense tells us that the physical damage created in an environment of high blood sugars occurs over time and involves several mechanisms. Any improvement in blood sugar control lessens damage. And when normalized, some existing damage appears to be reversible in some studies.

How long might it take for good control to reverse damage? The outlook as control is normalized may be similar to that of a person who stops smoking. After a smoker has stopped, it takes about seven years for the exsmoker's health risks to equal those of a nonsmoker. It is likely that for some of the physical damage caused by high blood sugars, a similar timetable holds for those who improve their blood sugar control. Although most damage cannot be reversed, a major benefit of attaining good control is that **it helps prevent further damage**.

How much damage can be reversed is unknown at this time, but reversal of damage is linked to the knowledge and effort applied. Early results on reversing kidney disease and neuropathy show great promise. In heart disease, the following interventions are making major impacts: using aspirin, antioxidants, chelated magnesium and B vitamins; reducing blood pressure, stress and dietary fat; and adding higher percentages of Omega-3 fatty acids to the diet.

The process remains complicated, however. Michael Brownlee, M.D., has proposed that glycosylation of proteins (see Chapter 20) can create permanently damaged by-products called Advanced Glycosylation Endproducts or AGEs. These glycosylated proteins may assume a life of their own with ongoing metabolic consequences and further health damage.[39] Dr. Brownlee is working with one promising chemical called aminoguanidine that appears to stop this unwanted glycosylation. But possible elevation of histamine, which can cause blood vessel leakage, in a few susceptible individuals, causes some caution in the use of aminoguanidine.[40]

Obviously, factors other than blood sugar control affect whether complications will occur. Still other factors affect the motivation to control blood sugars. The simple benefit of feeling better when blood sugars are stable and normal is often a more important motivation than what may occur in 5, 10 or 20 years. Chapter 20 looks at some mechanisms by which complications occur, and at interventions that promise to lessen damage, beyond the most important one of controlling blood sugars.

*"The great thing in this world is not so much where we are,
but in what direction we are moving."*

Oliver Wendell Holmes

PUMPING INSULIN

SAFE TECHNIQUES
FOR STARTING AND MAINTAINING A PUMP

4

These tips are provided to help you start on an insulin pump and continue to use it effectively.

BEFORE STARTING A PUMP

	Are you doing this now?	
• Do you test and record your blood sugars at least 4 times a day?[27]	yes**	no
• Do you use your blood sugar tests to adjust your insulin?	yes**	no
• Are you matching the carbohydrate in your meals to insulin intake by carbohydrate counting or the exchange system?	yes*	no
• Will you practice good sterile technique (washing, use of Betadine® Solution or Hibiclens® on the skin, etc.)?	yes**	no
• Are you a problem solver?	yes*	no
• Do you realize how important blood sugar control is to your health?	yes*	no
• Are you motivated to control your blood sugars?	yes**	no
• Do you have family and peer support?	yes	no
• Will you call your health provider if problems occur?	yes**	no

Your answers to these questions are ideally all "yes" **before** starting on a pump. Those marked with a single asterisk are **very helpful**; those marked with a double asterisk are **required**.

WHAT TRAINING DO YOU NEED?

Training is needed to manage an insulin pump well. Mastery of this material before starting a pump will be richly rewarded. You want to understand:

- how an insulin pump works (mechanics, programming, etc.),
- the timing and action of Regular insulin,
- how to count carbohydrates in your food to determine the amount of insulin needed for meals,
- how to chart and analyze your daily blood sugar tests,
- how basal rates and boluses are used,

- how to test basal rates, Carbohydrate Boluses and High Blood Sugar Boluses,
- what to do for low blood sugars,
- what to do for high blood sugars, and
- who to contact, and when, if problems should occur.

Some health care teams routinely put their patients in the hospital for pump start-up. You may find that this is the procedure your team uses. After starting on a pump, you'll need 24-hour telephone access to your physician/health provider team and your insulin pump manufacturer to deal with unanticipated problems.

Many experienced pump professionals recommend that bent metal needles be used for all pump starts. These infusion sets are very comfortable and provide greater certainty that insulin delivery is occurring. With a Sof-Set,® unless the insertion technique is exact, insulin delivery may be interrupted by a kinked teflon catheter. This kinking can cause variable blood sugars and at a pump start may not be recognized as the cause. Once blood sugar control has been achieved with bent metal needles, use of the Sof-Set® can be considered.

A Word To New Pump Users:

Unless your blood sugar control has been excellent before starting on a pump, the total insulin used each day with your pump will be less than what you're now using in your injections. High blood sugars create insulin-resistance. The improved metabolic control with a pump generally *lowers the need for insulin.*[41,42]

If you have any existing eye damage, even moderate background retinopathy, starting on a pump may cause *temporary worsening* for reasons that are not entirely clear. Some researchers believe a rise in insulin-like growth factors or the sudden lowering of glucose supplies is responsible. You'll want to have your eyes checked closely for this *transient worsening of retinopathy.*[43,44]

If your blood sugar control has not been great and you have retinopathy, your physician may advise that you improve your control gradually. With existing retinopathy, you want to be followed by an experienced ophthalmologist as you begin using your pump to ensure that eye changes do not progress during this period. After the first few months, expect retinopathy to stabilize and possibly improve, but see your ophthalmologist to verify this.

Supplies

Insulin:
Novo Nordisk™ Velosulin® Human Regular [45,46]
Reservoir or syringe:
Specific to each pump
Infusion set:
42" Polyethylene or Polyurethane tubing with bent metal needle or Sof-Set®
Disinfectant for infusion site:
Betadine® Solution or Hibiclens®
Adhesive material:
Micropore® tape, High Performance Tegaderm®, Silk tape, Polyskin®, or Opsite®
(Skin Prep® is a useful skin preparation for those with allergies to tape, etc.)
Blood sugar testing equipment:
Meter, strips, lancets, lancing device, charts

Low blood sugar treatment:
   Glucagon injection kit, glucose tablets, Sweet Tarts® or other dextrose candy, Monojel®

TO PREPARE THE RESERVOIR AND INFUSION SET

1. Pump reservoirs are coated with a lubricant to provide a tight seal between the O-rings and the barrel of the reservoir. If the reservoir has been sitting in a pharmacy for some time, the lubricant may pool inside the reservoir. To recoat the wall of a reservoir with lubricant, free the plunger and push it completely into the barrel. Rotate the plunger a couple of times to recoat the O-rings; then pull it back and forth twice in the reservoir to recoat the barrel. This spreads the lubricant onto the reservoir wall and O-rings for a good seal to prevent leaking of insulin between the O-rings.
2. Be careful to move the plunger straight back and forth in the reservoir. **Don't bend or wiggle the plunger relative to the reservoir barrel** as this can break the O-ring seal.
3. **If your reservoir is plastic, don't squeeze its barrel** as this may break the seal with the O-rings. Always hold the reservoir at the hub, especially for maneuvers requiring force, as when tightening the infusion set to the hub.
4. Fill the reservoir with Velosulin® human Regular insulin kept at room temperature.
5. To rid the reservoir of air bubbles, hold the reservoir in the palm of your hand and point the needle up with the air bubble toward you. Tip the reservoir so the bottom (plunger) end is slightly farther away than the needle end. Flick the reservoir with a fingernail or pen until the air bubble enters the neck of the reservoir. Then squirt insulin into the insulin bottle to get rid of the air bubble.
6. Air bubbles are harmless, but they do replace insulin. If air bubbles are noted in the infusion line, **an inch of air in the line is equal to half a unit of insulin**. In most cases, an inch or less of air in the line is not of concern.
7. Detach the needle from the reservoir. **Immediately** attach the infusion set to the reservoir while holding the reservoir at the hub.
8. The hub is a potential site for leaks. Be sure that the connection between the infusion set and the reservoir has been **firmly tightened**.

1" = 1 unit

9. **Manually prime the infusion line with insulin**.
10. Look closely **between** the O-rings for any sign of an insulin leak. Replace the reservoir if any liquid, mist or bubbles are noted. A leak between the O-rings may seem like a small amount of insulin, but it is enough to upset effective control.
11. Place the reservoir in the pump. Give 2 unit boluses until insulin is coming from the needle.
12. You are now ready to prepare the site and insert the needle.

SITE SELECTION

   The abdomen is the preferred site for the infusion set due to the rapid but consistent insulin uptake from this site. This steadier uptake of insulin from the abdomen lessens fluctuations in blood insulin levels and improves blood sugar control.[47,48] Great variations in insulin uptake can occur when insulin is injected into or near muscle sites, especially when exercise occurs. Insulin absorption from the abdomen, in contrast, is more consistent from day to day even with exercise.[49] Four or more abdominal sites are needed for rotation purposes.

To Prepare the Site

1. Wash your hands with soap and water.
2. Avoid touching the reservoir needle, the tip of the reservoir, the end of the infusion set or the top of the insulin bottle.
3. Hold your insulin bottle, reservoir, and infusion set up **away from your nose**. Don't breath or blow directly on the pump, the reservoir, the infusion set or the infusion site, as this is the cause for many skin infections. If you have had a history of minor skin infections in the past, you may want to obtain a surgical mask to wear over your nose and mouth to decrease the risk for infections.
4. Scrub the infusion site with an antiseptic solution. Use 1% or 2% iodine (Betadine® Solution) or chlorhexidine (Hibiclens®) to cleanse a site two inches in diameter on the skin. Iodine occasionally causes skin irritation in some people. If it does, wipe it from the skin with alcohol once it has dried to reduce this risk.

To Insert The Needle*

1. Insert a prebent needle into the skin at the prepared site. Position the needle so the metal attached to the plastic line is horizontal (i.e., pointing left or right from the navel, not up or down).

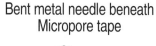
Bent metal needle beneath
Micropore tape

2. Apply a 3" length of 1/2" or 1" sized Micropore® tape or a sterile dressing such as Tegaderm HP®, Polyskin® or Opsite® directly over the needle. Place a second piece of tape over the needle at an angle to the first. But before pressing down the end of this second piece of tape, put a loop in the infusion line and place it under the end of the second piece of tape. This safety loop prevents the infusion set from being dislodged should the infusion line be accidentally pulled.

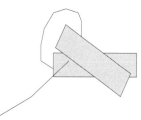

Navel

3. **Change the infusion site every 48 hours** to prevent a skin infection or abscess that requires an antibiotic or surgery.
4. **Check the infusion site daily** for redness, swelling or bleeding. Change the infusion site immediately if any of these occur.
5. Inspect the site for problems if your blood sugars are high.

* Sof-Sets® require special instructions, such as giving a 0.5 unit bolus to prime the line after insertion. Have a qualified instructor demonstrate how to insert these sets.

Rules For Reusing Bent Metal Needles

While it is not recommended, reusing bent metal needles is sometimes done to save money or protect the environment. If the choice is made to reuse needles, the skin site **must be changed every 48 hours** to prevent infections. Whenever needles are reused, **there is a greater chance for an infection**. Reuse bent metal needles with caution and at your own risk. Consult your physician/health care team regarding this. If a needle is reused, **sterile technique must be followed**:

1. Fill the reservoir full before the first use. **Never refill a reservoir** as the risks for leaking, clogging and infection are too great if the reservoir is refilled.
2. After 48 hours, remove the infusion set. Then remove the old Micropore® tape or other adhesive material from the infusion set.
3. Place the pump on the edge of a counter and place the infusion line under it so the needle hangs free in the air and does not touch anything.
4. Use a Betadine® swab to coat the last 3 inches of infusion line, including the needle. Then use the swab to coat and sterilize the skin at the new infusion site.
5. After the Betadine® Solution has dried on the infusion set, remove it with an alcohol swab.
6. After the alcohol dries on the infusion set, run a one unit bolus through the line to remove any Betadine® Solution or alcohol which may have gotten into the infusion needle.
7. Insert the sterilized infusion needle into the new infusion site and apply adhesive material.

What To Do:

For showers and bathing:

Clamp the infusion line and remove the reservoir from the pump. Be sure to clamp the line. If you don't, you stand a chance of giving yourself an accidental bolus of insulin. Put the pump in a dry area. Hang the infusion set around your neck (42" line), shower or bathe, and replace the reservoir in the pump afterwards.

Or leave the reservoir in the pump. Put the pump, even if waterproof, in a plastic bag or in a velcro camping bag to keep it dry. Or put the pump outside the tub or shower.

For sleeping:

Place the pump free on the bed, under a pillow, in a pajama pocket, or clamped to shorts or a soft belt.

For sex:

If you and your partner are comfortable with the pump, let the pump take care of itself in a convenient location. Women may want to attach the pump to a garter belt with the belt clip. As alternatives, clamp and remove the reservoir but leave the needle in place, or remove the infusion set entirely for a period of time no longer than 90 minutes. **Be sure to replace and restart the pump before falling asleep.**

FOR GOING OFF THE PUMP:

Occasionally you may want or need to discontinue pump use for a short period. Reasons for this may be a pump problem, an infection at the infusion site, a day at the beach, contact sport activities, or sexual relations. Table 4.1 provides instructions for maintaining control while off the pump.

How To Go Off Your Pump Temporarily	
How Long Will You Be Off?	**What You Need To Do:**
Less than 1.5 hours.	Nothing if BG is OK. A bolus is needed if BG is high or CHO will be eaten.
1.5-5 hours	Before disconnecting, take a bolus to cover 80% of the basal during the time off the pump. Cover CHO with injections.
Daytime Hours	Take an injection of Regular before each meal. Dose = CHO coverage + all basal insulin needed until the next meal.
Overnight	Take an injection of Lente or NPH at bedtime. Dose = 1.5 X basal needed during 8 hours of sleep.

Table 4.1 Going Off Your Pump

SITE INFECTIONS

Sterile technique and good hygiene are the best insurance against infections.[50] To prevent an infection, it is critical to follow the steps in "To Prepare The Site" on page 22.

If inflammation occurs in spite of this hygiene, change the infusion site. This inflamed site should not be used again until the inflammation and swelling have cleared. Call your physician if the inflamed site is larger than a dime. A topical antibiotic cream will often slow or prevent further spread of the infection if used early. If an infection is present, the reservoir and infusion set **must be removed and discarded**. Injected insulin should be used until an oral antibiotic has been started and the site checked. **Do not use the pump until the infection has been cleared.** Until it has been treated, an infection can spread to a new site.

Nonfatal toxic shock has been reported from infusion site infections in at least two pumpers: one was a noncompliant teenager, the other was compliant to instructions that used only alcohol as a disinfectant and allowed 72 hours (48 hours recommended) between infusion site changes.[51] **Always treat site infections with the utmost care.** If you are prone to skin infections, you may want to discuss with your physician having a broad spectrum antibiotic on hand for early treatment of a site infection.

ONGOING TIPS

High blood sugars can be a very serious problem. Any time your blood sugar readings are over 250 twice in a row without a good reason, replace your syringe and infusion set immediately. Take a conventional injection of Regular insulin and test your blood sugar often to make sure you are correcting the problem.

Do not continue to use your pump if your blood sugars remain high. If you are unable to correct a high blood sugar while using your pump, **stop using it**. Whenever two consecutive unexplained blood sugars occur, begin taking your insulin by injection. (The Velosulin® buffered Regular works fine for this.) Check your urine for ketones and call your physician/health care team immediately if ketones are present at moderate or large levels.

24

HbA1c or fructosamine levels should be checked every few months to assist in evaluating your overall blood sugar control. Remember that the HbA1c and fructosamine cannot detect erratic blood sugars nor replace frequent home monitoring.[52]

Always clamp the infusion line before removing the reservoir from your pump. Never prime the infusion set, nor attempt to free a clogged infusion line while you have the infusion set in place. These actions create a great risk of accidentally injecting a large dose of insulin.

Rarely, Velosulin® insulin that has been diluted may be needed by someone with very low insulin requirements. This is especially true for those taking less than 20 total units a day or in those using a basal rate of 0.4 units or less per hour. Use diluted insulin only if repeated clogging occurs on a low basal rate, or if your total daily insulin dose is so small that dilution becomes necessary in order to deliver these very small doses. The improved blood sugar control resulting from more exact insulin delivery can sometimes offset a slightly increased rate of clogging found with diluted insulin.[53]

Diluent for Velosulin may be obtained from Novo Nordisk™. A ratio of 1 to 1, insulin to diluent, is easy to work with. The pump then **remains set for use with U-100 insulin**, but the amount of insulin delivered by the pump is **actually half of the amount shown on the pump.** That is, a basal rate of 0.7 u/hr now delivers 0.35 u/hr, and a bolus of 7.0 units delivers only 3.5 units of the diluted insulin.

If a pump problem occurs, such as a leak, clog, or displaced infusion set, or if the pump is removed, the Regular insulin infused from a pump will be completely gone in 4 to 6 hours. ***Ketoacidosis can occur rapidly.*** Ketoacidosis can be especially dangerous if it occurs at night because an infusion set became displaced at bedtime. **It is recommended that you change your infusion set in the morning** rather than the evening. Normal daytime blood sugar monitoring can quickly pick up any problem with insulin delivery. Use careful technique at all times.

"Good judgement comes from experience;
and experience, well, that comes from bad judgement."

Anon.

ADVANCED WORKSHOP CHARTING

5

Normal blood sugars come from having insulin enter the bloodstream in the correct amount and at the correct time to balance other factors that raise or lower blood sugars (carbohydrates, activity, stress, etc.). Charting your blood sugars on Advanced Workshop Charts is an excellent way to collect information about the factors that affect your control. By using this information, you gain control. This chapter shows:

- why information is collected,
- how to put it on the Advanced Workshop Chart, and
- a sample Advanced Workshop Chart that has been filled in and analyzed.

GATHERING DATA

Charts tell you at a glance whether your blood sugars are above or below your desired range and the time of day problems seem to occur. They give you a clear picture of the details affecting your blood sugar control. When these details are visible on the charts, they can be analyzed to see what causes blood sugars to change. As the **reasons** for control problems are identified, **the tools in this book can be used to correct them**. Over time, charts tell you if you are getting where you want to go. They become your guide, letting you know if the changes you make are helping you gain better control.

One of the most important things to look for in charts is the pattern or trend of your readings. A pattern is any **consistent** rise or fall in blood sugars. It may be that you have frequent lows in the late afternoon, that your readings are simply running high most of the time, that eating a certain meal or eating out at a particular restaurant causes your blood sugars to go high or low, or that stress or changes in weight affect your readings. As you gather your chart information, patterns like these become apparent. Some typical blood sugar patterns and what to do about them are revealed in Chapters 17, 18 and 19.

The accuracy and details in your charts make it easier to rapidly adjust insulin for health. But with a busy schedule, you may let several days slip by while recording little information or none at all. And things never stay the same. Days lengthen and shorten, activity increases and decreases, weekends differ from weekdays, food intake shifts from more carbohydrate in the summer to more fat in the winter. All of these affect insulin need and blood sugar levels. Completed charts allow you to identify when and where insulin adjustments are needed.

The discipline required in charting leads to freedom from the worry of unknown internal damage, freedom from the annoyance of testing blood sugars that are always out of control, and freedom from the roller coaster mood swings that high and low blood sugars create. Most importantly, you gain the freedom to eat, work and exercise the way you want.

WHAT DO I PUT ON MY CHARTS?

The more information you place on your charts, the easier it becomes to control your blood sugars. Particularly important are blood sugar readings, carbohydrate intake, insulin doses and periods of exercise. Keep the chart, a small notebook or a data monitoring device handy for quick access. Most people find charting easier if they carry their chart with them.

A blank Advanced Workshop Chart is included at the end of the book. This chart was adapted for pump users by Reid Wronski from a chart originally developed by Katharine Alling in 1979. Use one of the two blank charts for practice. Carry this chart to the nearest copy store (with our permission and encouragement) to make plenty of copies for use. Begin charting your data to get a sense of how your blood sugars and the events of your life interact. To identify patterns and problem areas, record the following on your Advanced Workshop Charts:

BASIC INFORMATION

In the upper left hand corner, chart **your name, the date and the day of the week**. These identify who the charts belong to, determine if changes in blood sugar patterns are related to days of the week, and allow correct sequencing when laying the charts side by side to look for blood sugar patterns. Optional items like weight changes that affect insulin doses can also be recorded.

ACTIVITY

Record physical activity, exercise and work in the **activity area** near the top of the graph. Record any activity greater than your usual daily activity and any unusual activities. For instance, if you golf only on Saturdays this would be recorded. Occasional activities like this often have to be balanced with extra carbohydrate or a reduction in insulin doses. On the other hand, if you run 5 miles every day, this is normal daily activity for you and probably requires no change in your usual daily routine. If you don't run when you usually do, record that.

Rank your extra physical activity on a 1 to 5 scale. A "1" indicates a **mild** increase in activity. Give a "5" to activities that are **strenuous**. For instance, if sitting behind a desk is your usual work activity, but you spend the day moving your files and records to a new office, you would record a "1," "3," or "5" during the workday hours, based on how much work this moving required.

If you begin a running program and become quite winded on starting this new exercise, you would graph a "5" on your chart at the time this running took place. After you run for a few days or weeks, this same run may no longer be strenuous for you and would be listed as a "4" or a "3."

For more precise estimates of the carbohydrate intake and insulin adjustments for exercise, see Chapter 14. An example of charting physical activities is given in Figure 5.1.

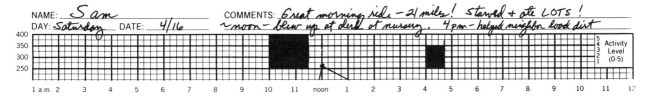

Figure 5.1 Activity Levels: This person bicycled for an hour and a half (level 5) in the morning, and then helped a neighbor load dirt into a trailer (level 4) for 45 minutes that afternoon.

BLOOD SUGAR RESULTS

Graphing blood sugar results provides a picture that lets blood sugar patterns be seen and dealt with. The minimum number of tests needed to adjust insulin doses is four a day: before each meal and at bedtime. Extra information is gained by testing 2 to 3 hours after meals. For a complete picture, seven tests a day are recommended to identify and analyze blood sugar patterns. Occasionally, a test at 2 a.m. or 3 a.m. is also needed. The boxes in the middle of the chart just below the blood sugar graphing area are for recording **blood sugar readings** and **insulin reactions**.

Test your blood sugar whenever low blood sugar symptoms occur, unless the symptoms are severe enough that waiting to test would be dangerous. If severe symptoms occur, test as quickly as possible after eating or ask someone else to test you. It's important to check your blood sugar if you feel low. Other conditions, such as excitement, fatigue, stress or anxiety can mimic the symptoms of a low blood sugar. An exact blood sugar measurement also allows you to take precise corrective action. Record all reactions to identify which insulin doses need to be lowered.

The time of all insulin reactions should be marked on the charts regardless of whether a blood sugar test was done. Indicate all verified and suspected insulin reactions on the chart with a circle or an arrow. It helps also to record the severity of the reaction. For instance, if symptoms are mild, use a small circle or arrow. If severe, use a large circle or arrow.

The first step in good blood sugar control is eliminating severe or frequent insulin reactions. Identifying the pattern in which they occur makes prevention possible. Be sure to also record on your chart any food eaten for a low blood sugar.

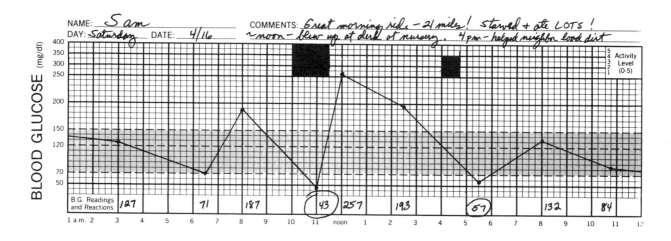

Figure 5.2 Graphed Test Results with blood sugars and insulin reactions noted at the bottom. Reactions with symptoms (circled blood sugars) are shown at 10:30 a.m. and at 5:30 p.m.

INSULIN DOSES

On the lines in the middle of your chart, record your **basal rates** and the timing of all **boluses**. Three lines exist for the three types of insulin doses: basal rate(s), Carbohydrate Boluses, and High Blood Sugar Boluses.

If your basal rate changes during the day, mark when this change occurs. Chapters 7, 8 and 9 present information on adjusting basal rates. Record Carbohydrate Bolus, the insulin used to cover carbohydrates in food (Chapter 10), on the line by that name when you take them.

28

At times, high blood sugars occur for which you need to take High Blood Sugar Boluses. A High Blood Sugar Bolus (Chapter 11) is the additional insulin used to lower high blood sugars. Figure 5.3 shows a sample of one day's insulin doses.

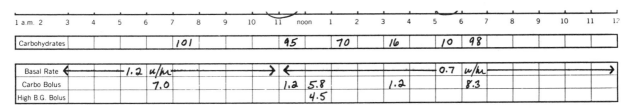

	1 a.m.	2	3	4	5	6	7	8	9	10	11	noon	1	2	3	4	5	6	7	8	9	10	11	12
Carbohydrates							101					95		70		16		10	98					
Basal Rate				1.2 u/hr													0.7 u/hr							
Carbo Bolus				7.0							1.2	5.8			1.2			8.3						
High B.G. Bolus												4.5												

Figure 5.3 Insulin Doses

FOOD LIST AND CARBOHYDRATE CONTENT

Carbohydrate is the main component in food that raises the blood sugar. Counting carbohydrates directly from a label or indirectly by measuring food exchanges is relatively easy to do. It also makes sense. For the first time, you are measuring **the part of food that influences your blood sugars**.

Chapter 6 shows how to identify and measure carbohydrates and gives instructions on how to determine your ideal daily carbohydrate intake. Measure and record all the carbohydrates you eat. Consult with your dietician at this stage for a precise recommendation of your own carbohydrate need, along with individualized information on ways to improve your blood sugars and health through your food choices.

The total daily carbohydrate intake recommended by your dietician can be broken into the number of grams you'd like to eat for each meal and snack during the day. The amount of carbohydrate you want at each meal can be tailored to fit your own schedule and food preferences.

At the bottom of the chart, clearly identify every food eaten, the time it is eaten, and the amount of carbohydrate it contains. Figure 5.4 shows an example. Be specific. A general word like "cereal" won't do. All cereals are not equal. Cheerios®, Grape Nuts®, Cornflakes®, and oatmeal can have very different effects on blood sugars. List precisely the type and amount of carbohydrate each food you eat contains. Writing "sandwich" down is very different from "sandwich: whole wheat/tuna/mayo, 32 grams." This is also very different from "sandwich: ice cream, 68 grams."

Only by listing exactly what you eat and the exact amount of carbohydrate the food contains can you determine what effect these foods are having on your blood sugars. You will find some foods have undesirable effects while others thought to be "bad" may be perfectly fine.

Don't overlook what you eat for low blood sugars. If you don't record the 4 graham crackers (44 grams) and 16 ounces of milk (24 grams) that you took for a nighttime reaction, you won't be able to determine why your blood sugar was 307 mg/dl in the morning.

List all foods, not just carbohydrates. You may discover that foods with little carbohydrate, like cheese or nuts, have a subtle effect and cause your blood sugar to climb gradually for several hours after you eat them. It helps if you also estimate how much of these noncarbohydrate foods you've eaten. List the amounts, like 2 ounces of cheese or 10 ounces of prime rib, on your charts.

BREAKFAST			LUNCH			DINNER		
Time	Food Description	Carbo's (gms)	Time	Food Description	Carbo's (gms)	Time	Food Description	Carbo's (gms)
7:00	nonfat milk 1 cup	13	1:00	nonfat milk	13	6:00	pasta with clam sauce	64
	Cheerios 56 grams	40		tuna sandwich	34		green salad	11
	rye toast x 2	30		apple 154 grams	23		glass of Chardonnay	6
	applebutter	8			70		vanilla ice cream	17
	strawberries	10						98
	poached egg	0						
		101						
MORNING SNACKS			AFTERNOON SNACKS			EVENING SNACKS		
11:00	blueberry muffin x 2	70	3:00	cheese	4			
	banana	25		crackers	12			
	diet soda	0						
		95	5:00	glucose tablets	10			

Figure 5.4 Food List and Carbohydrate Content

COMMENTS

In the **comments section** at the top, record any information you feel is relevant to your number data. Emotions, stress and illness can all affect blood sugars. This information might be "I have a cold," or "I woke up with a headache, may have had a reaction during the night." The high blood sugar before dinner could be explained by a comment that work was very stressful that day.

Emotions and blood sugars exist on a two-way street, and understanding these connections can help in your blood sugar control. The brain controls the secretion of various stress hormones which interfere with insulin. The brain, however, depends entirely on blood sugar for fuel. When high or low levels of sugar reach the brain, the response can be loss of memory, anger, irritability, slowed thinking or depression. Depression is common with high blood sugars. When depressed, a person has less energy to do the things needed for good control: thoughtful selection of foods, regular exercise and rest. And as blood sugars rise, hormones that prevent depression are lowered. The Comments section is the place to begin connecting your own emotions and blood sugars. Figure 5.5 shows an example.

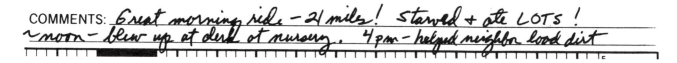

Figure 5.5 Comments

BLOOD SUGAR PATTERNS

As you place completed charts side by side, patterns of high and low blood sugars become evident. Set aside a time each week to look for patterns. For instance, every Saturday morning lay the last seven days' charts side by side.. Observe patterns including the time of day when high blood sugars or insulin reactions occur, drops in blood sugars due to exercise, high or low blood sugars following particular foods, high blood sugars following insulin reactions, and differences between weekend and workday blood sugars. Chapter 17 contains some typical blood sugar patterns and information on how to deal with them.

Be sure to show your charts to others. Listen to the suggestions of family and friends. Diabetes personnel have expertise in understanding the complexities of diabetes as it relates to daily life. Seek out this knowledge to shorten and simplify your path toward normal blood sugars. Another person, especially someone trained in diabetes care, will often see things that you miss. If you have any uncertainty about a potential pattern or the need to adjust your insulin, be sure to contact your physician/health care team for advice. Use these specialists to make your pump work for you.

The data collected in the Advanced Workshop Charts is more extensive than normally needed. However, by charting as many things as possible that influence your blood sugar control, you can begin to understand and change these factors. You can then use these same tools in the future, should you choose not to chart this extensively.

A SAMPLE CHART

On the next page is a complete chart for Sam, our sample pumper. An analysis of his chart is given below. Read Sam's background information below, but before looking at the analysis, examine his chart carefully. Make your own decisions about what you would change if you were Sam and this were your chart. What is happening to his blood sugars? Are they out of the normal range? If so, why? What would you do about it? You may want to write your suggestions down on paper for how to improve his blood sugars. After giving Sam's chart some thought about any changes you would make, look at the analysis that follows for confirmation of your thinking. Don't peek!

SAM'S BACKGROUND:

Sam has been using an insulin pump for 7 months. He weighs 151 pounds and leads an active lifestyle. He eats 2200 calories a day, with 1100 of these calories coming from carbohydrates. Usually he eats 275 grams of carbohydrate, with 80 grams for breakfast, 95 for lunch and afternoon snack, and 100 for dinner.

He uses one unit of Regular for each 12 grams of carbohydrate in his meals, having determined this ratio in previous testing (Chapter 10). When he has a high blood sugar, he takes 1 unit of Regular for every 30 points above 100 before meals (Chapter 11). He uses glucose tablets or Sweet Tarts® for his insulin reactions.

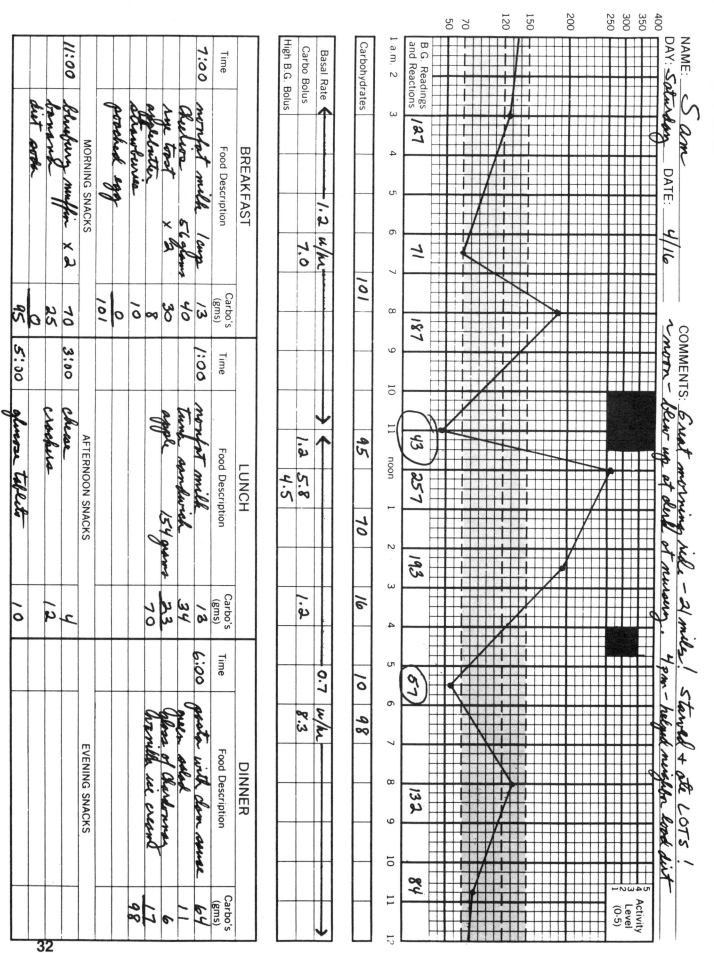

BLOOD GLUCOSE (mg/dl)

NAME: Sam
DAY: Saturday   DATE: 4/16

COMMENTS: Great morning ride — 21 miles! Started + ate LOTS! ~noon~ Blew up at Dink at noon. 4pm ~ helped neighbor load dirt

Activity Level (0-5): 5 4 3 2 1

	1 a.m.	2	3	4	5	6	7	8	9	10	11	noon	1	2	3	4	5	6	7	8	9	10	11	12
B.G. Readings and Reactions			127			71		187			43	257	193		16		57	98		133		84		
Carbohydrates							101				45	70	16		10		98							
Carbo Bolus											1.2 5.8						8.3							
Basal Rate	1.2 u/hr →						→				← 4.5				0.7 u/hr									
High B.G. Bolus																								

BREAKFAST

Time: 7:00

Food Description	Carbo's (gms)
nonfat milk 1 cup	13
Ovaltine 56 grams	40
rye toast x 2	30
applebutter	8
clementine	10
poached egg	0
	101

MORNING SNACKS

Time: 11:00

	Carbo's
blueberry muffin x 2	70
banana	35
diet soda	0
	95

LUNCH

Time: 1:00

Food Description	Carbo's (gms)
nonfat milk	13
tuna sandwich	34
apple 134 grams	23
	70

AFTERNOON SNACKS

Time: 3:00

	Carbo's
cheese	4
crackers	12

Time: 5:00

glucose tablets	10

DINNER

Time: 6:00

Food Description	Carbo's (gms)
pasta with clam sauce	64
green salad	11
glass of Chardonnay	6
vanilla ice cream	17
	98

EVENING SNACKS

ANALYSIS:

When you look at Sam's chart, you can see his blood sugar control was fairly good this day. Because it's a weekend, and the length and intensity of his activity is different than on a weekday, Sam has been testing his blood sugars more frequently than usual. His blood sugar readings average in the normal range and are reasonably steady through the day, with the first and last sugars absolutely normal. Five of eight blood sugar tests are out of the desired range.

Sam's basal rate of 1.2 units per hour between 3 a.m. and 11 a.m. is higher than during the rest of his day, probably to offset a Dawn Phenomenon (see Chapters 8 and 18). This rate, however, appears to be too high. His blood sugar dropped from 127 mg/dl at 3 a.m. to 71 mg/dl at 6:30 a.m. at this setting.

Sam's meals are generally good with balanced foods and a high carbohydrate, moderate protein, low fat intake. He took 7.0 units 30 minutes before breakfast. Since he uses 1 unit for each 12 grams, this would normally cover 84 grams of carbohydrate. He actually ate 101 grams, probably intending the extra 17 grams to help offset his bike ride later that morning. The blood sugar reading at 8 a.m. of 187 mg/dl an hour after breakfast reflects this lower than usual meal coverage.

On his bike ride, Sam rode 21 miles in an hour and a half at an average speed of 14 miles per hour. From Table 14.5 in Chapter 14, this level of exercise would use a maximum of 70 grams of carbohydrate each hour, or 105 grams for the whole bike ride. The extra 17 grams eaten at breakfast was not enough to cover this need.

The reaction at 11 a.m. resulted from this lack of carbohydrate and the excess morning basal insulin may have contributed as well. When the reaction occurred, Sam realized he had made an error. Unfortunately, the two blueberry muffins and banana he ate, on top of the stress hormones released by the insulin reaction (a large circle indicates this was a major reaction), caused his blood sugar to rise sharply to 257 mg/dl. When his ravenous appetite subsided and he realized he had overeaten, he partially corrected the excess carbohydrate with a 1.2 unit bolus, enough to cover 15 or so grams.

In his comments, Sam notes that he "blew up" at a nursery clerk at 11:30 that morning. The clerk may have deserved this response, but it's interesting that the incident occurred as Sam's blood sugar was spiking to the mid-200 range. This sort of irritability can occur at higher blood sugars or when blood sugars are low.

At lunch, he took a high blood sugar bolus to lower his blood sugar because it was higher than his target value. He wanted to be at 100 mg/dl, so he subtracted 100 from 257 to get his desired drop of 157. Since he drops 30 points per unit, he would normally take an extra 5.2 units in addition to his meal bolus. But he took only 4.4 extra units to bring the blood sugar down because much of the 1.2 units he'd just taken was still working. This appears to have been working well, as indicated by the drop in his blood sugar to 193 two hours after lunch.

He had an afternoon snack and covered it with an appropriate dose of insulin. Helping his neighbor shovel dirt into a trailer was not planned. Sam did not eat extra food nor reduce his insulin before starting to shovel. He covered the mild low blood sugar that resulted at 5:30 with 10 grams of glucose tablets, enough to raise his blood sugar about 40 points. Dinner was covered well with excellent readings 2 hours after dinner (132) and again at bedtime (84).

RECOMMENDATIONS FOR SAM:

- Think about reducing the morning basal rate (3 a.m. to 11 a.m.) from 1.2 units/hr to 1.1. Test this rate on another night to see if it needs to be reduced.
- Before increased activities like cycling or shovelling dirt, guesstimate more accurately the carbohydrate needed to cover them. Before the bike ride or a half hour into the ride, a banana along with a cup of milk could have been eaten (approximately 37 grams total), along with another 40 grams or so of carbohydrate fluids during the ride. From the chart, this 77 grams along with the extra 17 grams taken at breakfast probably would have covered the ride. (105 grams = maximum need)
- Take blood sugar tests before, during and after exercise or strenuous work. These are especially helpful for control of blood sugars.
- Note the relationship between irritability and blood sugars. If such a pattern exists and is recognized, it may avoid some embarrassing personal encounters.
- Always use glucose tablets first for reactions. They raise the blood sugar quickly and by doing so decrease the amount of stress hormones released. They also allow more rational decisions to be made on the quantities and types of foods used for reactions. See Chapter 13 for information on dealing with insulin reactions.
- Eat a bedtime snack when more activity than usual occurs. Extra physical activity can lower the blood sugar for 24 hours or more. Recognizing the extended blood sugar-lowering effect of exercise and that the night basal rate was too high could have prevented the reaction that happened early Sunday morning (not shown on this chart).

As you fill out the Advanced Workshop Charts, you may at first have some difficulty in recording all the information. However, by starting with good recording habits, you'll find it much easier to correct any problems you may run into on your pump. With practice, charting becomes a small distraction through the day.

Be sure to get in the habit of reviewing your charts regularly for patterns, as well as sharing them with your physician/health care team. We analyzed only one chart here due to space restrictions, but you will usually put a week's work--7 charts--side by side to analyze for patterns. Analyzing your charts encourages recognition and improvement of blood sugar patterns, keeps blood sugars as normal as possible, and maximizes good health.

"Take notes on the spot, a note is worth a cart-load of recollections."

Ralph Waldo Emerson

PUMPING INSULIN

CARBOHYDRATE COUNTING:
MANAGING YOUR NUTRITION

BY BETTY BRACKENRIDGE, M.S., R.D., C.D.E.

6

The insulin pump is the best tool now available to control diabetes and allow a free lifestyle. To get the most out of those advantages, however, you need a meal planning approach that's both as exact and as flexible as your pump.

Counting the grams of carbohydrate in what you eat is the most precise and flexible meal planning approach available, especially for those with Type I diabetes. To make the deal sweeter, it's also easier to learn and use than the traditional exchange system. Some people with diabetes use the exchange system or other approaches for dietary control. If you're currently on a pump and following one of those other meal planning systems, but are able to reach your blood sugar goals with that approach, by all means keep it up. But if your blood sugar control is not what you'd hoped for or you're interested in a more flexible and logical approach, consider carb counting.

The exchange system is based on **estimated** average nutrient values for a class of foods. Therefore, it is less exact than actually counting the grams of carbohydrate in each specific food you're eating. The imprecision in an exchange meal plan may be overlooked when using injections if insulin is not carefully adjusted and matched to food intake. But on a pump, the small, exact amounts of insulin delivered are best matched with a precise count of carbohydrate intake. If you're not using any meal plan system, definitely try counting carbohydrates.

This chapter describes:

- how the carbohydrate in food affects insulin need,
- how to calculate your daily need for carbohydrate,
- which foods have carbohydrate and how to count them,
- how to create a healthy meal plan based on carb counting, and
- the "bigger picture" in healthy eating.

WHY COUNT CARBOHYDRATES?

All foods, except pure alcohol, contribute glucose to the bloodstream. But the contributions are not equal. Fats have almost no direct effect on blood sugars and can largely be ignored. Only when an excess of certain fats are eaten can they block insulin action, making blood sugars rise more than expected after some fatty meals. Around 40% to 50% of protein intake ends up as blood sugar; however, the glucose from protein breakdown appears in the blood over several hours after a meal. Consuming average amounts of protein usually has little effect on blood sugars.

In contrast, 90% to 100% of the calories from digestible carbohydrates (starches and sugars) end up as glucose. This glucose enters the bloodstream shortly after eating. Therefore, the amount of insulin needed to cover a meal or snack can be closely estimated by simply counting the grams of carbohydrate that meal contains.

WHERE'S THE CARBOHYDRATE?

Before counting carbs, you need to know which foods contain them. Carbohydrates are found in varying amounts in the following foods:

- all fruits and vegetables,
- all grain products, such as breads, rice, cereals, potatoes and pasta,
- dried or canned beans, peas, nuts, and seeds,
- dairy products, particularly milk and yogurt, and
- beers and wines.

And though you might not eat them often, remember the high carbohydrate content of "splurge" foods like ice cream, cake, pie and candy. With carbohydrate counting, you can learn to handle **occasional splurges** so that they don't destroy your hard-won diabetes control.

FINDING THE CARBOHYDRATE CONTENT OF FOODS

Like height is measured in inches, carbohydrates are measured in grams. A gram is a unit used to measure the weight of very small items. There are about 28 grams in an ounce. But simply weighing a food does not tell how much carbohydrate it has. For example, a cup of milk weighs 224 grams, 2 graham cracker squares weigh 14 grams, and a tablespoon of table sugar weighs 12 grams. **But all contain the same amount of carbohydrate:** 12 grams. Although their total weights are different, these three food items will require the **same Carbohydrate Bolus** to cover them because they each have 12 grams of carbohydrate. You'll learn in Chapter 10 how much bolus insulin to take based on how many grams of carbohydrate you plan to eat.

To count carbohydrates, you'll need **information on the carbohydrate content of foods** (nutrition labels, food composition books, or food exchange lists) and **measuring equipment** (a digital gram scale, measuring spoons and cup). These are described in greater detail below.

Like any new skill, counting grams of carbohydrate will take some time and effort, especially at first. You'll need to weigh and measure foods for a while. This will allow you to "train your eye" to accurately estimate serving sizes and weights, especially when eating out.

Eventually, you'll be able to look at a piece of fruit, a plate of pasta or a combination plate in your favorite restaurant and quickly estimate their carbohydrate counts accurately, without weighing, measuring or looking up a thing. Be patient with yourself. It will take some time, practice and experimentation to develop that much skill. When you can precisely adjust your boluses to match the carbohydrate you eat, it will be worth all the effort.

SOURCES OF INFORMATION

Food Labels: Most packaged and processed foods have Nutrition Information Labels. These product labels contain valuable nutrition information, including the numbers of calories, carbohydrate, protein, and fat in **one serving** of the food. Labels are ideal for carb counting because the grams of carbohydrate in a serving are given on the package. An example is on the right.

If you're eating an 8 ounce carton of Elsie's Lowfat Yogurt, you have all the information you need to calculate an insulin dose. The label tells you that an 8 ounce serving has 43 grams of carbohydrate. Armed with this information and knowing how many grams of carbohydrate are covered by one unit of insulin from Chapter 10, you can figure out the Carbohydrate Bolus that will cover this food. But if the serving you will actually eat is **different from the serving size listed on the package,** you will have to weigh or measure your **actual serving** and do some calculations. Different ways to do this are described in the pages that follow.

Food Composition Books: Carbohydrate counting can be aided by reference books found in the "Nutrition and Diet" section of your local bookstore or library. One of the best known references is *Food Value of Portions Commonly Used* by Pennington and Church (Harper Collins Publisher, $14.00). Two other highly recommended references are Corinne Netzer's *The Complete Book of Food Counts* (Dell Publishing, $5.99) and *The Diabetes Carbohydrate and Calorie Counter* by Annette Natow and JoAnn Heslin (Pocket Books, $5.99). Pocket-sized gram counters are often sold at the supermarket checkout counter. One example is *Barbara Krause's Guide To Carbohydrates* (New American Library, $1.85). Use these books to learn the grams of carbohydrate in restaurant foods, packaged foods that don't have nutrition labels, and fresh foods, such as fruits, that aren't labeled at all.

If you use convenience foods, a book like *Convenience Food Facts* by Arlene Monk (DCI/ChroniMed, $10.95) which gives the grams of carbohydrate in 1,500 popular brand name products, will help. If you eat out often in restaurants, The *Restaurant Companion* by Hope Warshaw (Surrey Books, $9.95) will be a big help. In addition, many restaurants have brochures describing the nutritional content of specific items on their menus.

Food composition books and brochures, just like nutrition labels, describe the amount of carbohydrate in a specific serving size of each food. You will still need to weigh or measure your actual serving, and then do the necessary calculations to learn how many grams of carbohydrate are contained in your serving.

Food Exchange Lists: Food exchange lists can be used to determine the **approximate number** of grams of carbohydrate in foods. If you already know the exchange values of certain foods, you can use that information as a starting point. If you have brochures or handouts on the exchange system, you may want to use these to supplement other sources of information. Here are two examples that show instances in which using exchanges to estimate carbohydrate might have different results:

Example 1: Apple juice, 1/2 cup = 1 Fruit exchange   = 15 grams of carb
Actual carb value   **= 15 grams of carb**

The values are the same, so there's no problem. But for some foods, the exchange value and the actual carb count are different.

Example 2: Grapefruit juice, 1/2 cup = 1 Fruit Exchange = 15 grams of carb
Actual carb value   **= 10 grams of carb**

On a single item, these differences between the exchange system value and the actual grams of carbohydrate usually won't be large enough to matter in estimating a Carbohydrate Bolus. But when the carbohydrate content of several items in a meal is estimated using exchanges, bigger differences can develop. When an imbalance occurs between the actual carbohydrate eaten and the bolus insulin used to cover it, a high or low blood sugar results. Let your blood sugars guide you. If you're using exchange values and your blood sugar control isn't what you hoped for, try gram counting. It may be that you need that extra measure of precision to achieve excellent blood sugar control. Remember that matching the carbohydrate in foods with the correct Carbohydrate Bolus makes up about half of day-to-day blood sugar control.

Measuring Equipment

Measuring cups and spoons measure volume. Scales measure weight. For some foods there is a **big** difference. Take the example of Cheerios®. **Ten ounces of Cheerios® by volume** (1 1/4 cups) is equal to **one ounce by weight** (28 grams). Be sure you're clear on whether measures are for volume or weight. Many nutrition labels and food composition tables give both types of measure.

Measuring Cups and Spoons: Accurate measuring cups and spoons are available in many different places and price ranges. Be sure to use glass containers that allow you to "sight" across the top of the liquid for liquids and measuring cups for which you scrape a knife across the top to get the exact measure for dry items such as cereal and rice.

Gram scales: Look for these features in a digital gram scale: weighs food in grams and is accurate within 1 or 2 grams. Look also for a tare feature that will zero out the weight of a container. This allows you to portion food directly into a serving bowl, and eliminates the hassle of weighing foods on a scale and then moving them into your bowl. If you are able to invest some additional money in an item that can save you a great deal of effort, look for a **computerized gram scale**. These scales have been preprogrammed with information about how much carbohydrate is contained in different foods. When you enter the name of a food and place it on the scale, the scale automatically calculates the grams of carbohydrate in the food being weighed.

Several brands are available, ranging in price from about $50 to almost $200. They can be found in gourmet and kitchen shops. Mail order suppliers, like Nasco (901 Janesville Ave.; Fort Atkinson, Wis. 53538-0901) have a variety of gram scales for sale. For example, Nasco carries the Pillsbury Digital Gram Scale, which measures up to 2000 grams in one gram increments, for about $60. Gram scales are also available by mail from some diabetes supply companies.

How To Calculate Gram Values

When you eat a food like fruit that has no label or a serving that's different in size from that on the label or in the food listing---and you don't have a computerized scale that does the work for you---you have to calculate the grams of carbohydrate in your serving. Different calculation methods will be useful under different circumstances or with different foods. Let's say, for example, that you plan to eat linguine with pesto sauce. You cook the linguine and put the noodles on your plate after zeroing the plate out on the gram scale. The portion you want to eat looks good to you when the gram scale reads 150 grams. In Appendix A, you find that cooked plain spaghetti has a carbohydrate factor of 0.26 or 26% carbohydrate by weight. You can then use Method 1 on the next page to find the grams of carbohydrate your portion contains.

Method 1:   **Use the weight and carbohydrate factor for a food**

Find the carbohydrate factor for a food in the carbohydrate factor list in Appendix A.
Multiply the weight of the food in grams by its Carbohydrate Factor.

> **EXAMPLE:**

Weight of linguine portion   =   150 grams
Carbohydrate factor for spaghetti =   X 0.26
                                39 grams of carbohydrate

So, 150 grams of spaghetti (linguine) contains about 39 grams of carbohydrate.

Method 2:   **Use grams of carb per weight from food label or composition book**

Let's say you want to eat more than a single serving of Uncle Bob's Creamy Wild Rice. Here you have a choice of using your gram scale or a measuring cup to determine how much carbohydrate you're eating. Let's use the gram scale first because this is the most accurate method. The label to the right shows Uncle Bob's nutrition label:

UNCLE BOB'S CREAMY WILD RICE NUTRITION INFORMATION PER SERVING	
SERVING SIZE	1/2 CUP COOKED RICE (WT **38 GRAMS**)
CALORIES	130
PROTEIN	4 GRAMS
CARBOHYDRATE	27 GRAMS
FAT	1 GRAM

> **EXAMPLE:**

$$\frac{? \text{ grams of carbo in your serving}}{93 \text{ grams of rice (wt of your serving)}} = \frac{27 \text{ grams of carb (carb in std. 1/2 cup serv.)}}{38 \text{ grams rice (wt of standard 1/2 cup serv.)}}$$

Amount you eat = (27 X 93) ÷ 38 = 66 grams of carbohydrate

So, 93 grams of Uncle Bob's Wild Rice by weight contains 66 grams of carbohydrate.

Note: If you have to convert ounces to grams to do your calculations, this is done by multiplying the portion size in ounces (wt) by 28 grams/oz. (Example: 8 oz. portion X 28 grams/oz. = 224 gram portion size).

Method 3, which follows, may be slightly less accurate than Methods 1 and 2. This is because volume measures are more likely to vary than weights, especially if, for instance, you stuff your measuring cup with rice in the example below.

Method 3:   **Use the carb value per volume from the label or food listing**

$$\frac{? \text{ grams of carb in your serving}}{1.25 \text{ cup (volume of your serving)}} = \frac{27 \text{ grams of carb (standard 1/2 cup serving)}}{1/2 \text{ (0.5) cup rice (volume of stand. serving)}}$$

Amount you eat = (1.25 cup X 27) ÷ 0.5 = 68 grams of carbohydrate

Using Method 3, 1.5 cups of Uncle Bob's Wild Rice contains 68 grams of carbohydrate.
Remember though, if your own cup was stuffed, there may be 80 or 90 grams actually eaten.

How To Find Out How Much Carbohydrate You Need Each Day

Your daily carbohydrate goal is based on how many total calories you need. A healthy diet gets most of its calories, normally 50% to 65%, from carbohydrates. A person who needs 2000 calories a day would get 1000 to 1300 of those calories from the carbohydrate in breads, grains, vegetables, fruits, low-fat milk, and so on. Since there are 4 calories in each gram of carbohydrate, a person eating 2000 calories per day would need about 250 to 325 (1000 cal/4 to 1300 cal/4) grams of carbohydrate. That number becomes the basis of a carb counting meal plan. The total amount of carbohydrate for the day is divided up among the meals and snacks a person normally eats. (Remember, on the pump, snacks are not generally needed, as they are on injection therapy. If your basal rate is accurately set, you now have the freedom to enjoy snacks **when you want**, not when the insulin says you must.)

In a healthy diet most of these carbohydrates will come from nutrient-dense foods like whole grains, fruits, legumes, vegetables, and nonfat or lowfat milk and yogurt. Nutrient-dense foods are ones that have a high volume of nutrients like vitamins, minerals, fiber and protein for their calorie content. The carbohydrates contained in candy and regular sodas are fine, except that they lack the other nutrients that your cells require to remain healthy and they can cause blood sugar spiking. The carbohydrates and other nutrients found in nutrient-dense foods like brown rice and broccoli give you the most health value per calorie.

How To Calculate Your Own Grams Of Carbohydrate

Follow the steps below to get an estimate of your daily calorie and carbohydrate needs. Consult a dietician for specific help.

Step 1: Find your desirable weight

To determine your total daily calorie needs, you first need to know your **desirable body weight**. You can check a weight chart or use the formulas that follow to get an estimate. **If you are satisfied with your present weight, use this as your goal weight.** Otherwise, use the formulas below.

Women: Allow 100 lbs. for 5 ft. of height and 5 lbs. for each additional inch.
Example: Estimated target weight of a 5' 5" woman is 100 lb. + (5 x 5") = 125 lb.

Men: Allow 106 lbs. for 5 ft. of height and 6 lbs. for each additional inch.
Example: Estimated target weight of a 5' 10" man is 106 lb. + (10 x 6 lb.) = 166 lb.

A person with a small frame may want to subtract 10% from the value they get, while a large-framed person may need to increase his or her value by 10%.

YOUR CALCULATIONS

Woman, Average Frame Size

100 lbs. + (5 x _____) = _____   (+ or - 10% for large or
              (inches over 5')   (goal weight)   small frame)

Man, Average Frame Size

106 lbs. + (6 x _____) = _____   (+ or - 10% for large or
              (inches over 5')   (goal weight)   small frame)

Step 2: Find your calorie factor for daily activity

Besides your weight, how many calories you need each day is affected by your level of activity. On an active day, more calories (and more carbohydrate) are needed, while on a less active day, fewer calories are needed. The table below gives a **calorie factor** for typical activity patterns. Pick a calorie factor for your **usual level of daily activity** from the following table.

Activity Level	Calorie Factor	
	Male	Female
Very Sedentary: Limited activity; slow walking; mostly sitting.	13	11.5
Sedentary: Activities involve mostly walking; recreational activities include bowling, fishing, or similar activities.	14	12.5
Moderately Active: Recreational activities include 18 hole golf, aerobic dancing, pleasure swimming or similar activities.	15	13.5
Active: Greater than 20 minutes of jogging, swimming, competitive tennis or similar activities more than 3 times per week.	16	14.5
Super Active: At least 1 hour of vigorous activity such as football, weight training, or full-court basketball 4 or more days per week.	17	15.5

For Your Calculations

Pick your calorie factor from the list on the previous page and enter it here:

My calorie factor = _____

Step 3: Estimate your daily calorie need

Determine your approximate daily calorie need by multiplying your desirable body weight found in Step 1 by your calorie factor found in Step 2. For example, an active woman whose weight is 124 lbs. needs about 1800 calories per day (124 x 14.5 = 1798).

Your Calculations:

_____ x _____ = _____
(my goal weight) (my calorie factor) (my total daily calorie need)

Note that blood sugars in Type I diabetes should never be controlled by limiting calories **below what your body actually needs**. The road to blood sugar control lies in **eating what you need and adjusting your insulin to handle that amount of food.** When your blood sugar is in good control, your body behaves just like it did before you had diabetes. If you eat too much, you gain weight. If you eat too little, you lose weight. Keep track of your weight and your appetite. These tell you whether you're actually eating the right amount of food for you.

Step 4: Determine your daily carbohydrate calories

Divide your total calories by 2. The number you get is the total number of calories from carbohydrate needed in your daily diet to give yourself 50% of your calories as carbohydrate.

Your Calculations:

_____ ÷ 2 = _____
(my total daily calorie need)   (my daily calories from carbohydrate)

Step 5: Calculate your daily carbohydrate grams

Finally, divide this number by 4. The number you get is the total number of grams of carbohydrate to include in your daily diet. So our 124 lb. woman with an active lifestyle has a carbohydrate goal of about 225 grams each day (1800 total calories/2 = 900 carbohydrate calories/ 4 = 225 grams of carbohydrate) for a 50% carbohydrate diet.

Your Calculations:

_____ ÷ 4 = _____
(my daily calories from carbohydrate)   (my total daily grams of carbohydrate)

The number you get from this last calculation is your recommended total daily carbohydrate intake. This level of intake is a recommendation, not a requirement. Most typical diets in the United States contain less carbohydrate than this. If you have been eating considerably less carbohydrate, you may have difficulty consuming this amount, especially at first.

One way to judge whether consuming this much carbohydrate will be difficult for you is to simply eat your usual meals for a few days, while keeping a record of how much carbohydrate you actually take in. If you find that you are eating significantly less carbohydrate than your recommended quota, increase what you are getting now by 10% as you reduce your fat and protein calories by the same amount. You can make additional small increases later if you like. But because carbohydrate plays such a major role in setting your insulin doses, it is best not to abruptly make a big change in how much carbohydrate you're eating.

Your total daily carbohydrate allowance (either the amount calculated above or a lower value based on your current intake) should be divided into the amounts that you prefer for each meal or snack. Here are some examples of how a 225 gram total daily carbohydrate allowance might be divided among meals and snacks. **The exact pattern you choose should be based on your personal preferences and needs.**

Example 1: Likes big breakfast, light dinner, and bedtime snack
Example 2: Eats light breakfast and likes snacks
Example 3: Carbohydrate divided evenly among meals, no snacks

Meal or Snack	Ex. 1	Ex. 2	Ex. 3
Breakfast	75 grams	30 grams	75 grams
AM Snack		15 grams	
Lunch	60 grams	45 grams	75 grams
PM Snack		30 grams	
Dinner	45 grams	75 grams	75 grams
HS Snack	45 grams	30 grams	

AN IMPORTANT NOTE WHEN STARTING THE PUMP

When your basal rate and boluses are first being set, it is important to be as consistent as possible in your carbohydrate intake. For instance, if you normally eat less when your blood sugar is elevated, we recommend that you not do this during your first few days or weeks on the pump while your basal rates and bolus ratios are being set. It is far easier to make the needed adjustments accurately if only one major variable (insulin doses) is changing, rather than two (insulin doses **and** carbohydrate intake).

CARBOHYDRATES AND THE GLYCEMIC INDEX

Though carbohydrate counting is a simple and effective way to control blood sugars, it's not a perfect system. Research and your own experience have probably shown you that not all carbohydrates are created equal when it comes to their effect on blood sugar.

One attempt to measure these differences is called a "glycemic index." Researchers have developed lists which rank foods according to their glycemic index or ability to raise blood sugar.

For example, 15 grams of carbohydrate from white potatoes raises blood sugars higher than an equal amount of carbohydrate from sweet potatoes or yams. Carbohydrate from Cornflakes® raises the blood sugar **more than an equal amount from table sugar**, while the carbohydrates from white and whole wheat bread have about the same effect on blood sugars.

These differences are caused chiefly by how rapidly the carbohydrates from these different foods are digested. It's easier to understand how this can affect the blood sugar by picturing the water behind a dam. If all the water in the dam is released into the river on a single day, the river will run high, causing a lot of damage as that large volume of water moves along; however, the same amount of water can be released slowly from the dam over a long period of time. If this is done, the water level in the river would remain low. In a similar way, low glycemic index foods release their glucose to the bloodstream slowly. In contrast, high glycemic index foods release their carbohydrate rapidly into the blood after a meal

The glycemic index in Appendix B gives you a good idea how a particular food may affect your blood sugar in the hours after you eat it. The differences, however, are not seen beyond 4 to 5 hours if you cover the grams of carbohydrate correctly with your meal boluses.

A food like Cornflakes® that has a high glycemic index may raise the blood sugar higher and quicker than All Bran® or old fashioned oatmeal, which are lower on the glycemic index. If you start with a blood sugar of 80 before breakfast, eat an equal number of grams of carbohydrate from each cereal and cover each with the same correct carbohydrate bolus, your sugar before lunch should be back to around 80 after eating any of these three cereals.

The only question remaining is whether the midmorning blood sugar produced by a high glycemic index food is too high for good control. If it is, you may want to prevent this rise:

1. by eating less of the higher glycemic index food with a smaller meal bolus,
2. by eating less with a snack later,
3. by adding fiber (such as switching from white toast to whole grain cereal) to the meal to slow down digestion and absorption, or
4. by taking your meal bolus earlier to match up better with the glucose profile.

The glycemic index, however, is not a precise tool. Although the relative differences between foods are known, the exact effect on your blood sugar at a given time can be changed by a number of factors. These factors impact how rapidly a food is digested or absorbed, such as the amounts of fat and protein in the meal, the amount and type of fiber the meal contains, how fast the meal is eaten, and even whether the carbohydrates are eaten raw or cooked.

In spite of all these factors, the glycemic index can still be a useful tool. Gather information about your own response to foods under various situations, using self-monitoring of blood glucose. Armed with this information, you can create your own personal glycemic index and become even more skilled at balancing your insulin needs with your carbohydrates.

THE BIGGER NUTRITION PICTURE

When you have mastered the art of carbohydrate counting, you will be an expert in how to balance your insulin and food intake to achieve blood sugar control. As important as it is, however, blood sugar control is not the only health concern affected by nutrition. Your **overall** health is dependent on eating a wide variety of nutrient-dense foods.

The **amount of fat** in your diet is important. A high intake of fat is associated with greater risk for heart disease, cancer and obesity. These serious health problems are even more important to people with diabetes than they are to others. Heart disease is twice as common in people who have diabetes as it is in the general population. Because of this, a fat intake of no more than 20% to 30% of total calories is recommended by the American Diabetes Association, the American Heart Association, and the American Dietetic Association.

For most people, this means cutting way back on the amount of fat added to foods (butter, margarine, sour cream, oils and shortening used for frying, etc.), and choosing low-fat protein foods (fish, skinless chicken, and skim dairy products including cheese, for example). A low protein diet has been shown to **slow the development and progression of diabetic kidney disease**. Keeping meat portions small is highly recommended.

After talking about reducing our intake of some of those greasy old favorites, it seems only fair to talk about a change in the diabetes diet that is good news. As most of us remember, the dietary harangue in the past was **"No Sugar!"** That taboo has been loosening in recent years as blood sugar testing has shown that it's possible to retain glycemic control when eating some "splurge foods" **if** we know how to account for their sometimes hefty carbohydrate content.

Sugar is no longer banned from coffee, nor jelly from toast, nor an occasional small piece of pie from the dinner table. It appears that it may, in fact, be healthier to have a small amount of applebutter (which has no fat in it) on your waffle, rather than the butter or margarine that were recommended in the past.

No one really benefits nutritionally from an excess of these high-calorie, low-nutrient foods, whether he or she has diabetes or not. But small amounts can add flavor to a diet and, if chosen wisely, can allow fattier foods to be avoided. Be careful though: **sugar almost always travels with fat**. For instance, a chocolate candy bar gets about **60% of its calories from fat!**

Whether you include some sugar-containing foods in your meals or not, the key to blood sugar control is to determine the amount of carbohydrate in your food and cover it with an appropriate amount of insulin. This balancing of carbohydrates with insulin is at least half of blood sugar control. These actions, together with a nutrient-rich, low-fat, low-protein diet, are vital parts of a healthy lifestyle for those with diabetes and those without.

"The waist is a terrible thing to mind."

Ziggy (Tom Wilson)

PUMPING INSULIN

OVERVIEW OF
BASALS AND BOLUSES

7

This chapter provides the information needed:

- to understand the importance of insulin levels,
- to understand why different basal patterns are necessary,
- to understand how to use Carbohydrate Boluses,
- to understand how to use High Blood Sugar Boluses, and
- to estimate starting basal rate(s) and boluses.

WHY IS THE INSULIN LEVEL IMPORTANT?

Insulin plays a major role in the creation, release and use of fuels. The beta cells in the normal pancreas deliver the right amount of insulin into the blood to activate glucose transport into fat, muscle and liver cells. At the same time, enough glucose must be left behind in the blood so the brain and nervous system receive fuel for their vital functions. Other hormones counterbalance insulin by releasing glucose from glycogen stores in the liver and muscles.

If a person with Type I diabetes does not give himself enough insulin, his blood sugar rises. With too little insulin, cells that depend on insulin can't take in enough glucose; they lack fuel and the person feels tired. Additional insulin has to be given. If there is too much insulin in the blood, cells that use insulin will take in too much glucose. This can lower the blood sugar too far, leaving the brain and nervous system without enough fuel to think clearly and maintain coordination.

Since the body requires fuel at all times, insulin must always be present in the bloodstream to regulate fuel. The normal pancreas delivers insulin to cover **two needs**:

- as a constant background flow, and
- in shorter spurts delivered rapidly to cover the carbohydrate absorbed from food.

Insulin delivery in a pump, though, helps meet **three needs** in diabetes:

- as a constant background flow (Basal Rate),
- as coverage for carbohydrate in food (Carbohydrate Boluses), and
- to lower high blood sugars when they occur (High Blood Sugar Boluses).

Compared to multiple injections, one of the great advantages of an insulin pump is its ability to cover these three needs**separately**. Because needs can be covered separately, each part of the control process on a pump can be tested for accuracy. This testing of basal rates and boluses can usually be completed within the first month of pump use.

An Overview For Setting Insulin Doses

The goal in pump usage is having blood sugars as normal as possible. To reach this goal, you will be setting your insulin doses in a series of seven steps found in this chapter and in Chapters 8, 10, 11, 12 and 14. For best results, follow these steps in the sequence given. You may want to review the PumpFormance Checklist in Chapter 2, or read the entire book for a better understanding of what you will be doing, and then return to Chapter 8 where the testing begins.

Here is how it works: **First**, you'll find your estimated starting basal rate in Table 7.1 found later in this chapter. Next, you'll test and reset, if necessary, your night basal rate in Chapter 8. You will know that your night basal is correct when you can keep your blood sugar level through the night. In other words, when your blood sugar remains close to the same reading from bedtime through the night, your basal rate is adjusted correctly. The **third** step, also covered in Chapter 8, gives you your correct day basal rate. Here, the ability to maintain a level daytime blood sugar while fasting shows that your day basal is correct.

For the **fourth** step, you'll want to know how to count the grams of carbohydrate in your meals. This is covered in Chapter 6. You'll then use this information in Chapter 10 as you determine exactly how much carbohydrate is covered by a unit of insulin. The ability to balance the carbohydrate in your meals with Carbohydrate Boluses allows you to eat meals without losing control of your blood sugars.

If you happen to end up with a high blood sugar, you can use the **fifth** step to get your blood sugars back to normal. Step 5, outlined in Chapter 11, helps you set up your own table for sliding scale or supplemental boluses. This table tells you the correct High Blood Sugar Bolus needed to return high blood sugars that may happen before or after meals back to normal.

The **sixth** step in Chapter 12 provides another piece of the puzzle. Here the Unused Insulin Rule is described. This rule gives an estimate for how much insulin is still working from previous boluses. This allows you to avoid giving too much insulin when boluses overlap.

Because exercise affects the blood sugar, extra carbohydrate or less insulin is needed when you're engaged in increased physical activity. Principles allowing good control to be maintained during exercise are covered in Chapter 14 as the **seventh** step.

Together, these seven steps provide the major tools needed to set insulin doses for blood sugar control on your pump. Let's look more closely at what basal and bolus insulin doses do before beginning to test them.

Basal Insulin

Cells need a background or basal insulin supply at all times to receive fuel. Insulin controls **glucose** entry into some cells, helps regulate production and release of **fats** as fuel, and helps some **amino acids** that create enzymes and structural proteins to enter cells. Of the total daily insulin supply, 40% to 50% is needed as basal insulin to control the flow of these three fuels.[54]

The basal rate on a pump delivers this background insulin needed to control the availability and use of the fuels when you're not eating. Under most circumstances, only minor basal rate adjustments are needed to balance the changing output of "counter-regulatory" or stress hormones. For example, most people require a small upward adjustment during the early morning hours to counteract the presence of a Dawn Phenomenon. Chapter 9 covers some of the reasons for changing basal rates.

When first starting on an insulin pump, a single basal rate is a good place to start. This single rate is then tested to determine whether it is correct and whether more than one rate is needed. If a Dawn Phenomenon is suspected or known before the test, a varied basal rate may be chosen for the initial test by your physician/health care team.

Because most people have a Dawn Phenomenon, most require more than one basal rate. Basal insulin delivery from a pump is superior to injections in controlling an early morning rise in blood sugar levels, both on waking[55] and into the early afternoon hours.[56] On average, an increase of 20% in the early morning basal rate is needed to offset a Dawn Phenomenon.[57] A change in basal rate for a Dawn Phenomenon may be as small as 0.1 unit/hour (u/hr), as in a rise from 0.6 u/hr in the middle of the night to 0.7 u/hr during the hours of 2 a.m. to 8 a.m. A large increase in basal rates **is rarely needed if a small increase is made early, usually at 1 or 2 a.m.**

Compared to boluses, basal insulin has a slower effect on blood sugars. A bolus begins to lower blood sugars in 20 or 30 minutes, but an increase in the basal rate is not seen for 90 to 180 minutes after the change was made, unless the change is large.[58] Due to this delay, changing basal rates does not work well for lowering high blood sugars.

Remember that **bolus insulin doses cannot be accurately determined until the basal rates have been correctly set**. For instance, if the basal rate is too high, no meal bolus might be needed to cover a snack or meal, or if a bolus is given for a meal, it would be less insulin than expected. With a high basal rate, if the blood sugar were 80 to 120 before a meal and the meal and meal boluses were skipped, low blood sugar symptoms would begin shortly afterward.

If the basal rate is too low, just the opposite happens. A person would require larger than normal meal boluses to cover meals, and when a meal and a meal bolus were skipped the blood sugar would climb as the hours passed. Your basal insulin has to be adjusted to your needs before you will be able to determine how much bolus insulin you need for meals.

The basal rate is correctly set when
the blood sugar remains level or drops slightly while fasting.

BOLUS INSULIN

When the basal rate is correctly set, **bolus insulin** serves the last two functions:

- Carbohydrate Boluses cover the carbohydrate in your meals, and
- High Blood Sugar Boluses lower high blood sugars.

CARBOHYDRATE BOLUSES

Whenever carbohydrates are eaten by a person with a normal pancreas, insulin is released directly into the bloodstream. This insulin release is rapid and precisely matched to the carbohydrate in the meal. Figure 7.1 illustrates insulin release into the bloodstream. The shaded area shows **basal insulin** being constantly released to handle background metabolism for someone who does not have a Dawn Phenomenon. The spikes of insulin above the basal insulin show **boluses of insulin** that are released into the bloodstream to cover the carbohydrate eaten in those meals.

Carbohydrate boluses on a pump mirror the way a normal pancreas works. The amount of carbohydrate eaten in a meal determines the amount of bolus insulin needed. **The more carbohydrate eaten, the larger the bolus used to cover it.**

However, there's a major difference; a pump does not deliver insulin directly into the bloodstream but instead into the subcutaneous tissue under the skin. Because of the delayed absorption this creates, it is important that carbohydrate or meal boluses be given well before the

48

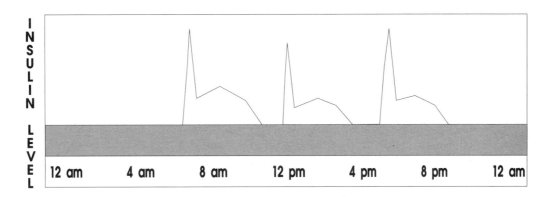

Figure 7.1 Normal Insulin Delivery into the Blood: Basal in grey and Boluses as after-meal spikes.

meal. Boluses for food work better when you give them **at least 30 minutes before a meal** if your blood sugar is normal. Carbohydrate from food breaks down quickly in the digestive tract and begins raising the blood sugar just a few minutes after eating. Compared to the pancreas' ability to deliver insulin directly into the blood, a pump bolus does not start to lower blood sugars until 30 to 90 minutes after it is taken. By giving more lead time for carbohydrate boluses to work, the spiking of blood sugars 1 to 2 hours after eating is reduced.

If your blood sugar is below 70 mg/dl, eat enough carbohydrate to raise your blood sugar to normal, and then take a bolus to match the amount of carbohydrate you will be eating. If your blood sugar is high and your schedule allows, it helps to take the meal bolus early along with the extra amount needed to lower your blood sugar. You may want to wait 60 to 90 minutes before eating, depending on the blood sugar reading. **Don't delay your eating any longer than you planned though, as this can cause a severe insulin reaction.**

You need a Carbohydrate Bolus every time you eat any carbohydrate, **except**:

- when correcting a low blood sugar with carbohydrate (see Chapter 13),
- or when compensating for extra physical activity with carbohydrate (see Chapter 14).

In Chapter 10, you'll determine how many grams of carbohydrate are covered by each unit of bolus insulin. Once you have determined this you can balance the carbohydrate in your meals and have normal blood sugars afterwards.

THE CARBOHYDRATE BOLUS IS CORRECTLY SET WHEN THE BLOOD SUGAR GOES FROM
70 TO 120 MG/DL BEFORE A MEAL TO 70 TO 120 MG/DL 4 TO 5 HOURS LATER.

HIGH BLOOD SUGAR BOLUSES

The higher your blood sugar is, the more High Blood Sugar Bolus insulin it will take to return your blood sugar to normal 4 to 5 hours later. Chapter 11 will show you how to determine **how many points your blood sugar drops on each unit of Regular insulin**. With this information, an individualized sliding scale can be created to give the correct bolus to lower any high blood sugar. Two scales are set up to cover high blood sugars: one for high blood sugars before meals and a second scale for high blood sugars between meals. Two scales are needed because the **target** for an ideal blood sugar changes: usually 70 to 120 mg/dl before meals and 140 to 180 mg/dl after meals. With these two sliding scales, you are ready to lower high blood sugars at any time of the day.

STARTING INSULIN DOSES

The first things to determine before starting a pump is how much insulin is needed in the basal rate(s) and boluses. Since only Regular insulin is used in a pump, and the way it is delivered differs from injections, the daily insulin need can only be estimated at first. Your physician/health care team will help you make this estimate of starting basals and boluses. Two guides are normally used to estimate your starting insulin doses on a pump:

• STANDARD FORMULAS BASED ON BODY WEIGHT

Standard formulas exist for estimating total insulin need based on weight. By plugging your weight into these formulas, your physician/health care team can closely estimate your daily insulin need.

These formulas give a close approximation of your total daily insulin dose; they don't reveal how much of this dose you'll need in your basal rate(s) and boluses, nor can they predict whether you will need one or more basal rate during the day.

Use the first column in Table 7.1 to find your weight. Then look at Columns 3, 4 and 5 to find the first estimate of your starting basal rate, the ratio of Regular to grams of carbohydrate in meals and the number of points your blood sugar is likely to drop per unit of Regular when high.

• YOUR PREVIOUS INSULIN DOSES

In the second column of Table 7.1, you can find the amount of insulin you have been using in the past with injections.

Your Weight (lbs)	Your Previous Average Total Daily Insulin Dose On Injections	Chapter 8 Starting Basal Rate (units/hr)	Chapter 10 Starting Carbohydrate Coverage: 1 unit bolus for each	Chapter 11 Starting High BG Coverage: 1 unit bolus for each
100	25 units	0.3 to 0.5	16 grams	60 pts >target
110	28 units	0.4 to 0.6	15 grams	54 pts >target
120	30 units	0.5 to 0.6	15 grams	50 pts >target
130	33 units	0.5 to 0.6	14 grams	45 pts >target
140	35 units	0.6 to 0.7	13 grams	43 pts >target
150	38 units	0.6 to 0.8	12 grams	39 pts >target
160	40 units	0.6 to 0.8	12 grams	37 pts >target
170	43 units	0.7 to 0.9	11 grams	35 pts >target
180	45 units	0.8 to 1.0	10 grams	33 pts >target
190	48 units	0.8 to 1.1	9 grams	31 pts >target
200	52 units	0.9 to 1.2	8 grams	29 pts >target
220	58 units	1.0 to 1.3	7 grams	26 pts >target
240	66 units	1.1 to 1.4	6 grams	23 pts >target

Table 7.1 **Estimates for starting basal rates and boluses based on either weight or the previous average daily insulin dose.**

This table gives only estimates of starting insulin doses. These estimates may not be appropriate for a given individual. Blood sugar tests, outlined in Pumping Insulin, have to be done to test for accuracy. Discuss this with your physician.

Simply add up how much insulin you normally use each day in your injections, including doses of both Regular and Lente, NPH or Ultralente. Then look for this number in the second column. Next look at Columns 3, 4 and 5 to find estimated starting basal rates and boluses based on your previous injected insulin doses.

If your blood sugars have previously been well-controlled on injections, the total dose of insulin you have been injecting each day will be very close to the total dose you'll need on a pump. If your control has not been optimal, your physician/health care team's experience with you and other pumpers will help them estimate the starting dose. These estimated basals and boluses are then tested and readjusted to match your actual need.

How To Determine Starting Basal Rates And Boluses

As noted, starting insulin doses can be determined from a person's weight or from their previous average daily insulin dose. Table 7.1 gives both ways for estimating starting doses. A person can find his or her weight in Column 1 of the table and then find the estimated basal rates and boluses for that weight in Columns 3, 4, and 5 (approximately. 0.1 u/lb/day or 0.22 u/kg/day as the estimated basal insulin need). Then they can locate the average total daily injected insulin dose in Column 2, and estimate insulin doses for a pump from this. If these estimated doses, based on weight and on previous insulin dose do not agree, **always start with the lower rate.**

Many factors, such as your food choices, activity, general health, age, sensitivity to insulin, and production of hormones that interfere with insulin's actions, affect your insulin need. If your weight is above your ideal body weight, you eat a high fat diet, exercise only at your desk, have been in poor control for some time, or produce more hormones that block insulin than the average person, you will need more insulin. If you're a teenager with high hormone levels aiding your growth, you will need much more insulin. Your physician/health care team's familiarity with these factors allows them to help you make accurate estimates of your basal and bolus requirements.

Using Table 7.1, fill in Table 7.2 to determine your own starting Basal Rate, Carbohydrate Bolus, and High Blood Sugar Bolus. If you are already on a pump, use this information to evaluate your current basal and bolus settings. If you suspect you need more than a single starting basal rate, be sure to discuss this with your physician/health care team. Be aware that the starting basal rate (and boluses) may need

Use Table 7.1 To Fill In The Blanks Below And Find Your Starting Basal Rate And Boluses			
Your Weight	_____ lbs		
Basal Rate Estimated From Your Weight		_____ u/hr	
Your Previous Average Total Daily Insulin Dose	_____ u/day		
Basal Rate Estimated From Your Previous Avg. Daily Insulin Dose		_____ u/hr	
Lower Of The Two Estimated Basal Rates			_____ u/hr
Lower of The Two Carbohydrate Bolus Ratios		1 unit of Reg. for each _____ grams of CHO	
Lower Of The Two High Blood Sugar Bolus Ratios		1 unit of Reg. for every _____ points over target	

Table 7.2 Estimates For Starting Basal Rate And Boluses, Based On Weight And On Previous Total Daily Insulin Dose Using Injections

to be reduced soon after starting on a pump, especially if your blood sugar control was previously poor. Improved blood sugar control often leads to a **decrease** in insulin resistance.[11,59] Testing this starting basal rate(s) is covered in the next chapter.

EXAMPLE

As an example, Frances weighs 160 pounds and is close to her ideal body weight. From column 1 in Table 7.1, her basal rate estimated from her weight would be between 0.6 and 0.8 units/hour. But while on injections she has had good control while taking 6 Regular and 30 NPH before breakfast, and 9 Regular and 5 NPH before dinner, for a total daily insulin dose of 50 units. From Column 2 in Table 7.1, her basal rate would be between 0.9 and 1.1 units/hour based on her previous average total daily insulin dose. Table 7.3 shows how she calculated her starting basal rate. Note that she chose a starting rate of 0.8 units/hour (higher end of the lower range, based on her weight), rather than 0.6 units/hour, because her control has previously been good on 50 units of insulin per day.

Example: How Frances Used Table 7.1 To Determine Her Starting Basal Rate And Boluses			
Frances' Weight	160 pounds		
Her Basal Rate Estimated From Her Weight		0.6-0.8 u/hr	
Her Previous Average Total Daily Insulin Dose	50 units/day		
Basal Rate Estimated From Her Previous Avg. Daily Insulin Dose		0.9-1.1 u/hr	
Lower Of The Two Estimated Basal Rates		0.8 u/hr	
Lower Of The Two Carbohydrate Bolus Ratios		1 unit of Reg. for each 12 grams of CHO	
Lower Of The Two High Blood Sugar Bolus Ratios		1 unit of Reg. for every 37 points over target	

Table 7.3 Estimate Of Starting Pump Doses For Frances

"Live more from imagination than from memory."

Stephen Covey

PUMPING INSULIN

SETTING AND TESTING BASAL RATES

8

Once your starting basal rate has been selected, test it for accuracy. The goal is to find a basal rate that will keep a normal blood sugar level or allow it to fall only slightly **when no food is eaten**. The testing is broken into different segments during the day for convenience. The times chosen for night and day basal tests match typical working and sleeping hours. Pumpers who work odd hours, a nightshift or varied shifts will need to adjust testing times to their own schedule.

Testing the **night basal** is done before the day tests because activities that affect blood sugars, like exercise and eating, are suspended during the night. Tests are repeated until the same desirable results are obtained two or more times at the same basal rate settings. When the correct night basal rate is determined, a normal waking blood sugar will be easy to achieve. It is then time for daytime testing.

Daytime basal tests are done in two segments to allow most meals to be eaten on test days. Typical testing involves conducting the first test of the day between waking and mid-afternoon. The second test of the day is done on another day from mid-afternoon to bedtime. The starting basal rate(s) is adjusted, if necessary, until one or more rates are found to keep the blood sugar stable through the entire day.

This chapter provides:

- sample basal rate patterns, and
- instructions for testing your own basal rates.

When first starting on an insulin pump, previous injections of insulin will remain in the bloodstream for several hours. Basal testing should be delayed until 36 hours after the last injection of Lente or NPH, or 72 hours after the last injection of Ultralente.

FIVE COMMON BASAL PATTERNS

An insulin pump works best when it delivers background insulin in a manner that mimics a normal pancreas. Examples of five common basal insulin patterns are shown in the figures that follow. These patterns show the variety of ways insulin, given as the basal rate, might be needed by different people during a 24-hour period when no food is eaten.

The patterns below are **only examples**. They are models for basal patterns and a place for you to start. **Your basal pattern may be quite different and must always be tested with the help of your physician and health care team.** A method to test your basal rates is provided later in this chapter.

The Constant Basal Pattern

A constant basal rate is a good place to start for many pumpers. This will satisfy insulin need in 30% to 40% of those who go on pumps and closely approximate need for perhaps another 30%. Figure 8.1 shows a constant basal pattern: a straight, level line indicating the need for insulin at a constant level through the entire day.

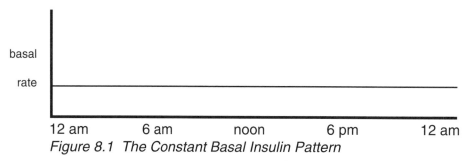

Figure 8.1 The Constant Basal Insulin Pattern

The Dawn Phenomenon Basal Pattern

Figure 8.2 shows the most common pattern, a basal rate for someone with a **Dawn Phenomenon**. **Between 50% and 70% of pumpers require extra basal insulin in the early morning hours to offset a Dawn Phenomenon.** The rise in the blood sugar between about 3 a.m. and 9 a.m. is caused by an increased release of growth hormone.[60] People who have a Dawn Phenomenon often raise their basal rate starting between 1 a.m. and 3 a.m. and then lower it between 9 a.m. and 11 a.m.

Why raise the basal rate so long before the blood sugar begins to rise? Because it takes 90 to 180 minutes for the blood insulin level to rise **after the basal rate has been raised**. At least a one to two hour lead time is needed to keep blood sugars from rising. Better blood sugar control results from a small basal rate increase at 1 a.m. or 2 a.m. than from a large one after the liver has already begun producing glucose around 3 a.m.

Before attempting to cover a Dawn Phenomenon, discuss this increased night basal rate carefully with your physician/health care team. Extra caution is required in raising nighttime basal rates due to the increased risk for low blood sugars. **Never assume you have a Dawn Phenomenon without first testing to see if you do.** Testing to determine whether you have a Dawn Phenomenon is covered later in this chapter. A typical basal pattern for someone with the Dawn Phenomenon looks like this:

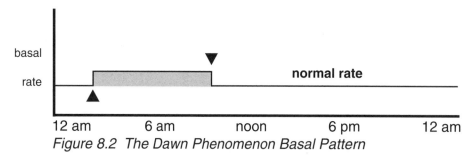

Figure 8.2 The Dawn Phenomenon Basal Pattern

Either the Constant Basal Pattern or the Dawn Phenomenon Basal Pattern will work for most pump users. But if blood sugars are not controlled with either of these, then try one of the other approaches, depending on the time of the day that blood sugars are poorly controlled. Be sure to test the pattern carefully.

The Nighttime Low Basal Pattern

Researchers have found that the lowest blood sugar of the day usually happens around 2 a.m. In one study of people on both conventional injections and multiple injections, researchers found that people with diabetes had a low blood sugar every fourth night on average.[61] People are most sensitive to insulin between midnight and 3 a.m. The liver seems to play a major role in this decreased need for insulin. The liver lowers its glucose production in the middle of the night and then increases production 2 to 4 hours before waking. This middle-of-the-night drop in the need for insulin requires that the basal rate be lowered at about 9 p.m., with a return to normal between 2 a.m. and 5 a.m. A basal rate pattern for someone (who does not have the Dawn Phenomenon) which lessens the risk for middle-of-the-night reactions looks like this:

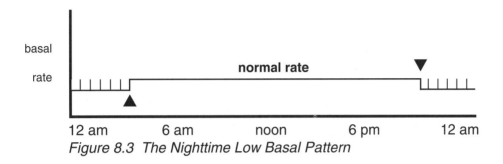

Figure 8.3 The Nighttime Low Basal Pattern

The Combined Nighttime Low/Dawn Phenomenon Pattern

Some pumpers require both less basal insulin during the night to avoid low blood sugars in the middle of the night, but a higher basal rate before waking for a Dawn Phenomenon. The basal rate is reduced at about 9 p.m., then raised above normal at 1 a.m. to 3 a.m. At 9 a.m. to 11 a.m., the basal rate is again lowered back to normal. A basal pattern to match this need is shown in Figure 8.4:

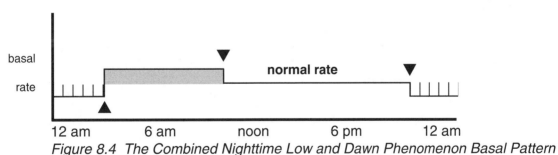

Figure 8.4 The Combined Nighttime Low and Dawn Phenomenon Basal Pattern

The Afternoon Low Basal Pattern

Figure 8.5 depicts another common pattern: a basal rate pattern to prevent low blood sugars in the afternoon. These afternoon low blood sugars often result from a buildup of insulin in the blood from boluses given earlier in the day for breakfast and lunch, combined with more physical activity during daytime hours. A lower basal rate starting between 10 a.m. and noon that returns to normal at about 4 p.m. to 6 p.m. can often prevent afternoon reactions. A smaller Carbohydrate Bolus for lunch can also be considered. This pattern looks like this:

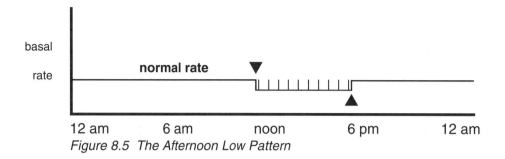
Figure 8.5 The Afternoon Low Pattern

Because of the precision and flexibility of insulin delivery with a pump, it is much easier to make these adjustments for changing insulin need during the day than it is with injections. Some pumpers, particularly those who exercise strenuously or for prolonged periods, find they benefit from 3 to 6 different basal rates each day to allow insulin levels to be lowered during exercise. Pumps that allow a temporary reduction in the basal rate are also convenient for exercise.

With experience, you will be making these changes as needed. Be sure to consult with your physician/health care team if you are uncertain what your results mean or you suspect that you need more than one basal rate during the day. The basal rate tests below will clarify what your own basal insulin needs are.

A Correct Basal Rate Is
The Most Important Step In Controlling Your Blood Sugars.

Steps To Test And Adjust The Night Basal Rate

In this section you'll take your estimated starting basal rate(s) from Table 7.2 in the last chapter and test it for accuracy. Once the night basal rate is accurately set, you can:

- go to bed with a normal blood sugar, eat little or no bedtime snack, and wake up with a normal blood sugar in the morning. (This is assuming your dinner bolus is no longer active and you've had no unusually strenuous activity that day.)
- safely correct any high bedtime blood sugars and wake up with a normal reading in the morning.
- rest peacefully. You, your spouse, parents, children, friends, roommates, and physician/ health care team will all sleep better knowing you're unlikely to have a reaction during the night.

Not only do you experience a full night of sound sleep, but your day starts better when you wake up with a normal blood sugar. Waking up during the night in the middle of an insulin reaction, or thirsty and tired from a high blood sugar, doesn't promote sound sleep. Having a steady blood sugar in a desirable range through the night is the first step to having normal readings through the day.

Don't try this test following a day in which you've had a severe insulin reaction, major emotional stress or unusually strenuous exercise. Major insulin reactions and excessive stress release stress hormones into the bloodstream that raise blood sugar levels for the next few hours.

56

Strenuous exercise can have just the opposite effect by enhancing insulin's action for several hours. Occurrences like these in the hours before your test can distort your results.

Follow the directions in Table 8.1 for the night basal test. Follow the suggested steps to prepare for the test, then test your blood sugar at the suggested times. (Testing times may need to be tailored to your own work and sleep hours.) Basal rates are then adjusted from the blood sugar results. Raise or lower the basal rate as instructed until the basal rate keeps your blood sugar relatively flat on at least two consecutive tests. Be certain to check with your physician/health care team before starting your test, or if you have any doubts about your doses, about how to interpret the readings, or whether to change the timing or level of your basal rate.

Don't forget the 2 a.m. test! This middle-of-the-night blood sugar is critical for determining whether and when the night basal rate needs to be increased or decreased, and whether more than one basal rate is needed. Once you have obtained desirable results on at least two occasions with the same basal settings, you'll be ready to test the day basal rate.

THE CORRECT NIGHT BASAL RATE KEEPS THE BLOOD SUGAR FROM RISING,
OR LOWERS THE BLOOD SUGAR NO MORE THAN **30** POINTS OVERNIGHT.

STEPS TO TEST AND ADJUST THE DAY BASAL RATE

Follow the directions for testing the day basal rate (First Part, then the Second Part) in Table 8.1. Test your day basal rate when nothing is interfering with your blood sugars, like a recent meal or a bolus of insulin that is still working. For these tests you'll want to start them either when you get up in the morning, or when at least 5 hours have passed since your last bolus and 3 hours after your last food was eaten. When you test at these times, only the basal rate will be affecting the blood sugars. Testing the day basal rate is done in two parts for convenience and accuracy. Fasting is required for the test. It's easier to fast only a half day rather than a whole day.

The first part of the test starts when you wake in the morning and ends in the mid-afternoon. Skip breakfast and have a late lunch. The second part of the test covers the late afternoon and evening. During this part, eat breakfast and an early lunch, but delay dinner until just before bed.

People often have reservations about skipping meals in order to test their basal rate(s). Some find it difficult to imagine going a few hours without food, but the human body is amazingly adaptive and will survive this ordeal. Some object: "They've always told me to eat when I take any insulin." The beauty of a pump is that this is **no longer necessary**. Remember, a correctly set basal rate is usually the most important step toward having normal blood sugars. A few hours of fasting is a small price to pay. If you are concerned about having a reaction on your current basal rate, check your blood sugar more often and consult with your physician/health care team about doing your test with a basal rate lower than your current setting.

Note that the blood sugar at the start of the test must be between 100 and 150 mg/dl. Although the upper point of this range is above that generally recommended, it allows room for the blood sugar to fall if the basal rate has been set too high. Once the basal rate is correctly set, ideal blood sugars can be more safely achieved and maintained.

For those who tested their night basal as suggested earlier in the chapter and found a single basal rate worked well overnight, the day basal rate is likely to be identical or very similar to this night rate. However, if your basal rate had to be increased in the early morning hours for the Dawn Phenomenon, one of the first things you'll need to determine is when during the morning hours this higher rate needs to be reduced.

Remember, the basal rate has to be reduced at least 2 hours before the blood sugar begins to fall. Because the extra insulin coming from a higher basal rate continues to work for 2 to 3 hours after the rate is lowered, the basal rate must be adjusted downward well before the blood sugar starts to drop in the afternoon. Similarly, if your basal pattern is the Nighttime Drop, the Combined Nighttime Drop/Dawn Phenomenon, or the Afternoon Drop, you have to determine when during the day to make the required changes in your basal rate.

Once the day basal rate is correctly set, you can:
- skip meals when necessary.
- eat meals late without the worry of a reaction.
- bolus precisely for carbohydrates and high blood sugars.

FIRST PART OF THE DAY BASAL TEST

Do this test on a day when you expect to be at your normal level of activity, as extra work or exercise will themselves lower the blood sugar. As in the previous test, there must be no strenuous exercise, no excess stress, nor a major insulin reaction in the hours preceding the test. Repeat the test until you have had the same desirable results on at least two occasions at the same basal rate settings.

SECOND PART OF THE DAY BASAL TEST

The second part of the day basal test covers the mid-afternoon to bedtime hours. Since you've already found the correct basal rates for the morning and early afternoon hours, and also the rate that starts the night basal, the basal rate for this part of the day fills in the remaining hours.

The basal rate for the test during the second half of the day is easy to determine from the rate already determined to end the first half of the day and from the basal rate that begins at night. For instance, if you found your morning/early afternoon rate to be 0.7 units/hour, the starting basal rate for the afternoon/early night will likely be between 0.6 and 0.8 units/hour. Check with your physician/health care team regarding the proper basal rate to begin the test. Test this rate until you have the same desirable results on two consecutive tests.

COMMENTS ON BASAL RATE TESTING

- Always consult with your physician/health care team to select your starting basal rate(s).
- For the first part of the day test, eat no breakfast and a late lunch, unless a low blood sugar occurs. For the second half, have an early lunch, start the test 5 hours after the lunch bolus, and eat dinner close to bedtime.
- Test your blood sugar often if you believe it may drop.
- If your blood sugar drops below 70 mg/dl, have at least 15 grams of carbohydrate and end the test. Discuss lowering your basal rate with your physician/health care team. If the drop in blood sugar is rapid, a major decrease in the basal rate is needed. If the drop occurs slowly, a small decrease is needed.
- If your blood sugar rises above 200 mg/dl, take a bolus to correct the high blood sugar and end the test. Discuss raising your basal rate with your physician/health care team. If this blood sugar rise is rapid, a major increase in the basal rate is needed. If the rise occurs slowly, a small increase is needed.

58

**YOU'RE SEEKING A BASAL RATE THAT MAKES YOUR BLOOD SUGAR
STAY LEVEL OR FALL NO MORE THAN 30 POINTS IN AN 8-HOUR PERIOD.**

With experience, you will be making these changes as needed. Be sure to consult with your physician/health care team if you are uncertain what your results mean or you suspect that you need more than one basal rate during the day.

**NEVER CHANGE THE BASAL RATE BASED ON ONE DAY'S BLOOD SUGARS
UNLESS DOING BASAL TESTING OR UNLESS THE RATE IS OBVIOUSLY INCORRECT.**

Basal Tests	How To Prepare For The Test	When To Test Blood Sugars	How To Readjust Basal Rates If The Test Fails (Blood Sugar Rises Or Falls)
Night Test	Take your dinner bolus at least 5 hours before bed. BG must be 100 to 150 at bedtime to start the test.	Bedtime, 2 AM, and on waking	If BG rises over 20 points during either bedtime to 2 AM, or during 2 AM to waking, raise basal rate during that period by 0.1 u/hr. If BG falls over 20 points in either period, lower the basal rate during that period by 0.1 u/hr. Retest.
First Part of Day Test (Waking to Mid-Afternoon)	No bolus for 5 hours and no eating for 3 hrs before start of test. BG must be 100 to 150 at start. (No breakfast and a late lunch.)	Every 1 to 2 hours	If BG rises more than 30 points during this period, raise basal by 0.1 u/hr and retest. If BG falls more than 30 points, lower basal by 0.1 u/hr and retest.
Second Part of Day Test (Mid-Afternoon to Bed)	No bolus for 5 hours and no eating for 3 hrs before start of test. BG must be 100 to 150 at start. (An early lunch and a late dinner.)	Every 1 to 2 hours	If BG rises more than 30 points during this period, raise basal by 0.1 u/hr and retest. If BG falls more than 30 points, lower basal by 0.1 u/hr and retest.

Table 8.1 How To Test Basal Rates

Cautions in Testing Basal Rates:
1) Test your blood sugar any time you feel it may be going high or low.
2) If your blood sugar drops between 70 and 100 mg/dl before a test starts, use glucose tablets to raise it. Five grams of glucose will raise the blood sugar 20 points. Retest in 20 minutes; start the test when over 100.
3) If stress hormones are released due to a low (shaking, sweating, excess hunger), cancel the test for that day.
4) If your blood sugar drops to less than 70 at any time, eat carbohydrate and end the test.
5) If your blood sugar goes above 200, take a bolus to correct the high blood sugar and end the test.

BASAL RATE TIPS:

- **Set and test the basal rates before testing boluses.** Basal insulin requirements have to be correctly set before carbohydrate or high blood sugar boluses can be determined.
- Most people benefit from having **more than one basal rate** a day, although the change in basal rates through the day is **usually small**.
- The best basal rate is one that causes the blood sugar to **stay constant or to drop slightly** over several hours while not eating. (Those whose basal rate may cause a slight drop in their blood sugar overnight should be sure to eat a bedtime snack. Carbohydrate will be needed when the bedtime blood sugar is less than 80 mg/dl to 100 mg/dl.)
- Change the basal rate **2 hours before** the blood sugar begins its rise or fall.
- With a Dawn Phenomenon, control is often better when the basal rate is raised by 0.1 to 0.2 u/hr at 1 a.m. or 2 a.m. than by a larger rise at 3 a.m. or 4 a.m.
- Signs that a basal rate is **too high**:
  Frequent lows during the night or before breakfast
  Frequent lows through the day
  Blood sugar drops when a meal is skipped
- Signs that a basal rate is **too low**:
  Frequent highs
  Blood sugar rises when a meal is skipped
- **Quick Basal Rate Check:** Does the daily basal insulin dose make up 40% to 50% of the total daily insulin dose?

"The cloning of humans is on most of the lists of things to worry about from science, along with behavior control, genetic engineering, transplanted heads, computer poetry and the unrestrained growth of plastic flowers."

Lewis Thomas

PUMPING INSULIN

WHEN TO CHANGE BASAL RATES

9

Under most circumstances, basal rates are not changed unless there's a clear reason to do so. Reasons to change the basal rate(s) can include exercise or activity that lasts several hours, or a vacation where activity is higher and stress levels lower than usual. Coverage for carbohydrates, corrections for high blood sugars and compensation for short periods of exercise are normally made by changing **boluses** rather than changing the basal rate. **But some situations demand that the basal rate (and boluses) be changed:**

CHANGE IN ACTIVITY LEVEL

Physical fitness affects sensitivity to insulin. Marathon runners, for example, are quite sensitive. They have about half as much insulin circulating in the blood as a person of the same height and weight who doesn't exercise heavily. When a person's level of physical activity increases, a lowering of the basal rate is often required.

If you work as a flight attendant and are going to spend two weeks bicycling in Canada, plan on a substantial reduction in your basal insulin requirements. Just the opposite happens if activity levels are lowered. If you had been working as a framer on a construction crew, but are now working at a desk as a project cost estimator, this decrease in activity is likely to increase your need for basal insulin.

The extra muscle activity and improved muscle tone brought about by activities like long-distance bicycling can greatly increase sensitivity to insulin. Longer, intense activities like this can require that insulin doses be rapidly lowered. As much as a 30% to 40% reduction in the basal rate may be needed at the start of such strenuous activity. Plan ahead for any major change in activity level. A quick call to your physician/health care team can prevent problems.

Lowering the basal rate is not needed for exercise that lasts less than 60 minutes unless it is quite strenuous. But for exercise that is moderate or strenuous in intensity and lasts longer than 60 to 90 minutes, a lowering of basal rates for a few hours is usually required. The basal rate(s) is lowered 90 to 120 minutes before the exercise begins and, depending on the exercise, kept at a lower level for 8 to 36 hours after it ends. See Chapter 14 for more information on adjustments for exercise.

CHANGE IN WEIGHT

Your bathroom scale is a quick guide to your basal rate. When you weigh more, you need more basal (and bolus) insulin. As your weight drops, your basal rate is reduced. Two factors play a role in how you set your basal rate during weight changes.

First is the **speed** of the weight change. If swimsuit season is suddenly upon you, or you decide at the last moment to attend your high school reunion, or out-of-town relatives call to tell you they'll be visiting next month, **weight-panic** often sets in. Where did those extra pounds come from and how can they be shed quickly? Eating may be quickly reduced in this concern over image.

This type of weight loss is not recommended. But if you decide to lose weight in this manner, be aware that your basal rate will need a quick reduction. A basal rate reduction of 10% to 30% may be needed after a few days if you suddenly restrict calorie intake. Boluses, of course, are also lowered in relation to how far you reduce your carbohydrate intake and to your increased sensitivity to insulin.

The second factor to be considered is the **amount of weight lost or gained**. A gradual change of 5 pounds or so may have little effect on the basal rate setting. If the shift is 10 pounds or more, an adjustment in the basal rate will likely be needed. **The greater the weight change and the faster the weight change, the more you need to change your basal rate.**

GASTROPARESIS

Gastroparesis is damage to the nerves that control the wave-like motion of the intestines. This loss of normal intestinal motion can cause food to be absorbed more slowly after a meal than normal, creating problems in blood sugar control because of this delay. When a person with gastroparesis gives a bolus to cover food, an insulin reaction often occurs 2 to 3 hours later, followed by a high blood sugar some 6 or 8 hours later. A person with gastroparesis may benefit from a higher than normal basal rate during the day to cover eating, with little or no meal boluses.

Most blood sugar problems have nothing to do with gastroparesis. Never blame your own control problems on gastroparesis without discussing this thoroughly with your physician.

HEAT, COLD, AND HEIGHTS

As temperatures change outside a home, the thermostat in the home's heating/air conditioning system responds by raising or lowering the temperature. As your utility bill will tell you, maintaining a constant temperature can require **lots of energy**. Your body acts the same way, using more glucose and fat as it warms or cools itself. The increased metabolic rate required to cool or heat the body uses additional energy that may lower the blood sugar. If you are outside in unusually hot or cold weather, slightly lower insulin doses may be needed. This is especially true in hot weather when the body uses more energy in cooling and sends more blood flow to the skin. The increased circulation picks up insulin faster from the infusion site and speeds up the action of insulin. A slightly lower basal rate may be required.

A similar circumstance occurs in changing to higher altitudes. More energy is required to breath and pump blood as the air becomes thinner. The resulting increase in metabolism is apparent in the first few days after arriving at a higher elevation. Until the body adapts, a lower basal rate or additional carbohydrate may be required.

ILLNESSES

Illnesses, especially bacterial infections, place extra stress on the body. Extra insulin as larger boluses or higher basal rates is often needed to fight this physical stress. During bacterial illnesses, like pneumonia, a strep throat, an impacted wisdom tooth, a bladder infection or a sinus

62

infection, more insulin will be needed, especially when illness is accompanied by a fever. Bacteria are usually more stressful to the body than viruses and can easily cause total insulin need to double. After an antibiotic has been started, however, **any temporary increase in basal rates or boluses will have to be quickly reduced to prevent insulin reactions**.

Illnesses that last several weeks, like hepatitis and mononucleosis, often require that basal rates and boluses be raised. Shorter viral illnesses, like a cold or flu, have more varied effects on blood sugars. When short-term viral illnesses occur, it is often easier to control blood sugars by using high blood sugar boluses as needed, rather than by raising the basal rate. These boluses may be needed even though eating is reduced. Always remember:

THE QUICKEST WAY TO LOWER A HIGH BLOOD SUGAR IS TO TAKE A BOLUS (NOT INCREASE THE BASAL RATE).

More insulin can be given quickly with a bolus than by increasing the basal rate. A bolus of 10 units takes only a few minutes to deliver. To get the same amount of insulin by increasing the basal rate would typically take 10 to 15 hours if the rate is doubled. The extra speed in insulin delivery from boluses can be critical during an illness. Boluses can be repeated every few hours as needed (see Chapter 12). Always remember to check that your pump is actually delivering insulin whenever blood sugars are unexpectedly high.

Illnesses that cause vomiting or diarrhea may not affect the basal rate. Reduced eating can usually be offset by reducing or eliminating boluses. However, if a bolus has been taken for a meal, but one is unable to eat or vomiting occurs, the basal rate may be lowered or suspended **temporarily** to reduce the chance of an insulin reaction. Intake of apple juice, regular 7-UP® or other quick sugar can also be helpful. Be certain to test your blood sugars often or have someone else test it for you during any illness.

MENSES

Many women find their blood sugar rises in the days just before their period begins. Sometimes this increase is small enough that it does not require changing the basal rate. Many women, however, will note a substantial increase in their need for basal and bolus insulin during the few days prior to their period.

Once a change in insulin requirement during menses has been determined and blood sugars are stabilized on a pump, the timing of monthly periods and the increased need for basal insulin become more regular and predictable. A similar change in basal rates can be expected at about the same time during your cycle in future months. If you observe a monthly change occurring, discuss it with your physician/health care team for a way to match it with a cyclic insulin adjustment.

MEDICATIONS

Certain drugs greatly increase the need for insulin. Paramount among these are steroids like prednisone and cortisone. Whether taken for poison ivy, for illnesses such as lupus or asthma, or as an injection into an inflamed joint, steroids generally make insulin need rise sharply. One of us (the one with diabetes) got a severe case of poison oak while clearing fire brush out of a field. This required prednisone tablets to be taken for a few days, which caused a substantial rise in blood sugars and insulin requirements. Basal rates were raised and larger boluses were taken, some of which were 4 and 5 times those normally used.

Occasionally, the physician who properly recommends the use of oral or injected steroids for medical problems may be unaware how dramatically they can affect blood sugar levels. Steroids injected into joints will usually increase insulin needs for 3 to 5 days. If steroids are required, make sure the physician prescribing them is aware of your diabetes. Contact your physician/health care team as soon as possible to discuss insulin adjustments that are likely to be needed.

POST-MEAL SPIKES

Many people notice that a couple of hours after eating, their blood sugars rise to very high levels. If the blood sugar remains high until the next meal, the solution is usually simple: either raise the Carbohydrate Bolus taken for the previous meal or lower the amount of carbohydrate in it. When the blood sugar spikes above a desired range (usually 150 to 180 mg/dl) between meals, however, and then returns to normal before the next meal, a more complicated problem exists. The meal bolus can't be raised or a low blood sugar will occur.

A common cause of spiking between meals is that the meal bolus was taken too close to the meal. Try taking the meal bolus earlier if this is the cause. But if the bolus was taken at an appropriate time and the food choices are good, the basal rate may be raised in combination with a reduction in the meal bolus. This can often reduce post-meal spikes. Again, the rise in basal rates is usually small, about 0.1 or 0.2 u/hr, and is started about 2 hours before the meal. Discuss this with your physician\health care team.

PREGNANCY

The greatest risk for ketoacidosis on a pump occurs overnight due to a mechanical failure, such as an infusion set that becomes displaced at bedtime or during the night. When ketoacidosis is to be strictly avoided, as it is during pregnancy, a combination of injected bedtime Lente or NPH, equal to 50% of the overnight basal, **plus a lower nighttime basal rate** greatly reduces the risk of morning ketoacidosis.[8] This technique uses the pump for controlling fasting blood sugars, and at the same time uses long-acting insulin given in an injection to prevent fasting ketoacidosis.

Insulin requirements gradually climb during pregnancy. During the last six months of pregnancy, Dr. Lois Jovanovic-Peterson, a specialist in diabetes and pregnancy, has found that basals and boluses need to be increased every 7 to 10 days.

"Quit worrying about your health. It'll go away."

Fletcher Knebel

Pumping Insulin

Setting And Testing
Carbohydrate Boluses

10

Boluses can be determined **only after the basal rate is correctly set**. Set and test your basal rate(s) before attempting to determine boluses. Boluses normally provide 50% to 60% of the total daily insulin dose. Boluses are used:

- to cover carbohydrates, and
- to lower high blood sugars when they occur.

Matching the carbohydrates in each meal with individualized Carbohydrate Boluses allows greater freedom in choosing foods and in the timing of meals and snacks. The correct ratio of insulin to carbohydrate is determined largely by how sensitive one is to insulin. Insulin sensitivity, in turn, is affected primarily by body weight and physical activity.

More weight and less physical activity correspond with less sensitivity to insulin. An overweight person who is **severely insulin-resistant** may require one unit of Regular for every 2 to 5 grams of carbohydrate. But a **thin, insulin-sensitive person** may use only one unit for every 20 grams. For most people with Type I diabetes, a unit of Regular is needed for every 8 to 16 grams of carbohydrate. Table 7.1 can be used to obtain a close estimate of your own ratio.

The ratio of insulin to carbohydrate may vary slightly for different meals during the day. A unit of Regular often covers less carbohydrate (fewer grams) at breakfast compared to other meals. Variation in sensitivity to insulin at different times of the day occurs for two reasons: counter-regulatory hormone levels change through the day (usually higher in the morning), and carbohydrate boluses taken earlier in the day affect blood sugars later that same day due to their prolonged action.[62]

Fuels That Affect The Blood Sugar

Three fuels in food can affect the blood sugar: carbohydrate, fat and protein. **Carbohydrates have the most impact on the blood sugar.** Because carbohydrate is so important, the insulin given for a meal is calculated to match its carbohydrate content. Carbohydrate counting is an excellent way to determine insulin need; however, any system that quantifies food, estimates insulin accordingly, and achieves good blood sugar control can be used.

High fat meals have some effect on blood sugars. Fat may delay the intestinal absorption of carbohydrate and reduce the usual rise in blood sugars after a meal.[63] On the other hand, a high fat meal may cause temporary insulin resistance.[64, 65] A high fat diet can lead over time to weight gain and insulin resistance, particularly in those prone to male pattern obesity.[66, 67] Insulin resistance involves changes in metabolism that makes it harder for sugar to be used as fuel, while at the same time more fat and sugar are produced and released into the bloodstream. **Insulin resistance is not**

good for health. Most effects of a higher fat diet are seen over the long run; only small effects on blood sugars are seen following a particular high fat meal.[68]

Protein in the diet is usually eaten in such small portions that its affect on the blood sugar is minimal.[69] Large quantities of protein in a meal, however, can have a more immediate effect on the blood sugar than fat, because 40% of protein calories are converted to glucose over a period of several hours. The amount of protein required to significantly raise blood sugars usually requires eating an 8 oz. steak or several ounces of cheese.

Following a high-protein dinner, for instance, blood sugars will rise slowly with the total impact usually not seen until the following morning. Bolusing for large amounts of protein in a meal is not recommended due to the slow onset and long duration of this protein effect. An increase in the basal rate may be considered for a few hours after **some high protein meals**.

HOW TO DETERMINE CARBOHYDRATE BOLUSES

Table 7.1 gives a quick guide to determine your starting ratio of Regular to grams of carbohydrate. Similar to basal rate determinations, the carbohydrate bolus ratio is based on weight or on previous average 24-hour injected insulin dose (whichever gives the lower bolus estimate). Once determined for normal circumstances, of course, carbohydrate boluses can be lowered as needed for exercise.

To determine carbohydrate boluses, the grams of carbohydrate in the meal you plan to eat is first counted. Carbohydrate counting is a simple way to optimize blood sugar control and is explained in Chapter 6 and Appendix A.

Although the correct ratio of a unit of Regular insulin to grams of carbohydrate is critical to good blood sugar control, another important factor is timing: **how long before a meal the bolus is given**. Because the pump is so convenient, someone using a pump may forget to take a meal bolus soon enough before a meal.

Your Weight (lbs)	Your Previous Average Total Daily Insulin Dose On Injections	Chapter 8 Starting Basal Rate (units/hr)	Chapter 10 Starting Carbohydrate Coverage: 1 unit bolus for each	Chapter 11 Starting High BG Coverage: 1 unit bolus for each
100	25 units	0.3 to 0.5	16 grams	60 pts >target
110	28 units	0.4 to 0.6	15 grams	54 pts >target
120	30 units	0.5 to 0.6	15 grams	50 pts >target
130	33 units	0.5 to 0.6	14 grams	45 pts >target
140	35 units	0.6 to 0.7	13 grams	43 pts >target
150	38 units	0.6 to 0.8	12 grams	39 pts >target
160	40 units	0.6 to 0.8	12 grams	37 pts >target
170	43 units	0.7 to 0.9	11 grams	35 pts >target
180	45 units	0.8 to 1.0	10 grams	33 pts >target
190	48 units	0.8 to 1.1	9 grams	31 pts >target
200	52 units	0.9 to 1.2	8 grams	29 pts >target
220	58 units	1.0 to 1.3	7 grams	26 pts >target
240	66 units	1.1 to 1.4	6 grams	23 pts >target

Table 7.1 Estimates for starting basal rates and boluses based on either weight or the previous average daily insulin dose.

This table gives only estimates of starting insulin doses. These estimates may not be appropriate for a given individual. Blood sugar tests, outlined in Pumping Insulin, have to be done to test for accuracy. Discuss this with your physician.

Boluses work best if given 30 to 45 minutes before eating, or earlier for high blood sugars.

But there are times when you can't give your bolus at the appropriate time before a meal. If you plan to eat out at a restaurant or you're in a situation where the timing of a meal is uncertain, you may not be able to give the full carbohydrate bolus 30 to 45 minutes before the meal. But you might consider a smaller bolus, say 1/4 to 1/2 of the total bolus that's anticipated for the meal. Then give the remaining bolus when eating actually starts and the carbohydrate count is more certain. This partial bolus allows the blood insulin level to begin rising, but reduces the risk of a low blood sugar. The same technique can be used if the timing of a meal is known but the amount of carbohydrate is not. **Fast-acting carbohydrates should always be available in case the blood sugar drops before the meal is actually served.**

TESTING CARBOHYDRATE BOLUSES

The Carbohydrate Bolus Test starts with an **estimated** ratio of Regular to grams of carbohydrate found in Table 7.1. Test this estimated ratio as shown in Table 10.1. As testing proceeds, adjust the starting ratio as needed until you find the correct ratio for your own needs.

A correct ratio returns the blood sugar to within 20 to 30 points of the original reading 5 hours after the meal. Test your blood sugars 2, 3 and 4 hours after eating to reduce the risk of hypoglycemia. Repeat the test several times to determine the most accurate ratio. Remember that slight variations in your ratio may occur for food eaten at different times during the day.

Time	Action
30 to 45 Minutes Before Meal	1. Test your blood sugar. 80 to 120 mg/dl is ideal to start the test. 70 to 150 is OK.
	2. Determine how many grams of carbohydrate (CHO) you will eat.
	3. From Table 7.1 and your physician's recommendations, decide how many grams of CHO are covered by 1 unit of Regular for you. Divide this number into the total number of grams of CHO you plan to eat. Take this insulin as a bolus if it seems OK.
At Mealtime	4. Eat the number of grams of CHO chosen in Step 2.
2 Hours After Meal	5. Test your blood sugar. a. If the blood sugar has risen 40 to 80 points above Step 1, this is OK. b. If the blood sugar has risen less than 40 points, too much insulin may have been given. Test more often to avoid an insulin reaction. c. If the blood sugar is over 240, END THE TEST and correct the high sugar.
3 and 4 Hours After Meal	6. Repeat Step 5.
5 Hours After Meal	7. Test your blood sugar. a. If within 20 to 30 points of your starting blood sugar in Step 1, this is probably the correct meal bolus ratio for you. Retest to verify. b. If more than 30 points above Step 1, start your next test with a smaller grams of CHO number (i.e., if you were using 1 unit for each 12 grams, go to 1 unit for 11 grams, thus increasing your meal bolus.). c. If more than 30 points below Step 1 or an insulin reaction occurred, start the next test with a larger grams of CHO number (i.e., if you were using 1 unit for each 12 grams, go to 1 unit for 13 grams, thus reducing your meal bolus).

Table 10.1 How To Test Carbohydrate Boluses

PUMPING INSULIN

SETTING AND TESTING
HIGH BLOOD SUGAR BOLUSES

11

HIGH BLOOD SUGAR BOLUSES

Besides covering carbohydrates, boluses are also used to lower high blood sugars. When high blood sugars occur, any physical damage that might result is lessened if the sugar is high for only a short period of time. But caution is necessary when lowering a high blood sugar to avoid an insulin reaction. To lower a high blood sugar safely, you need to know how many points your blood sugar drops for each unit of Regular insulin. Once this is known, you can set up a table that gives the number of units to take for readings that are high before or after meals.

To use a High Blood Sugar Bolus, first choose your target goals for before meals and for after meals. In other words, what blood sugars do you and your physician/health care team feel is safe and desirable before and after meals? Since blood sugars rise after eating, the target goal after a meal is higher than before a meal. For many pumpers, a target of 100 mg/dl before eating and 180 mg/dl two to three hours after eating is reasonable. These targets should be discussed with your physician/health care team and tailored to your own needs, such as pregnancy (lower target) or a history of hypoglycemia unawareness (higher target). This chapter covers:

- how to determine how far your blood sugar will drop on a single unit of Regular,
- how much High Blood Sugar Bolus to add to the Carbohydrate Bolus for premeal highs, and
- how much High Blood Sugar Bolus to take for highs that occur after eating.

Similar to Carbohydrate Boluses, the number of points the blood sugar drops for each unit of Regular depends on weight and sensitivity to insulin. These, in turn, are related to the total amount of insulin a person uses each day. The distance the blood sugar drops per unit of Regular stays the same unless infection, ketoacidosis, a marked change in physical activity, or other factors are present. If your blood sugar drop per unit of Regular **varies greatly from one time of day to another**, the basal rate should be retested for accuracy.

Table 7.1 on page 50 gives an estimate of the number of points the blood sugar will drop for each unit of Regular insulin based on the total daily insulin dose. The last column of this table is based on a formula using the "1500 Rule" developed by Paul C. Davidson, M.D., Medical Director of the Diabetes Treatment Center at HCA West Paces Ferry Hospital in Atlanta. The 1500 Rule states that the estimated drop in a person's blood sugar for each unit of Regular = 1500 ÷ their current total daily insulin dose.

A person can set up a personalized High Blood Sugar Bolus Table using this information. The amount of insulin you take for a high blood sugar is determined by how far the high blood sugar is above a selected target goal and by how far your blood sugar will drop on each unit of Regular. Your individualized scale shows how much insulin you need to take for high blood sugars at various readings above your target blood sugars before or after meals.

68

A High Blood Sugar Bolus is usually needed for every high blood sugar occurring before a meal. This bolus is added to the normal Carbohydrate Bolus for the food in the meal. However, you may not need a High Blood Sugar Bolus if you plan to exercise after the meal, and the exercise will lower the high blood sugar.

| Blood Sugar Reading (mg/dl) | High Blood Sugar Bolus Needed: | |
	Before A Meal	After A Meal
100-119	0	0
120-139	0.5 unit	0
140-159	1.0 unit	0
160-179	1.5 units	0
180-199	2.0 units	0
200-219	2.5 units	0.5 unit
220-239	3.0 units	1.0 unit
240-259	3.5 units	1.5 units
260-279	4.0 units	2.0 units
280-299	4.5 units	2.5 units
300-319	5.0 units	3.0 units
320-339	5.5 units	3.5 units
340-359	6.0 units	4.0 units
360-379	6.5 units	4.5 units
380-399	7.0 units	5.0 units

Table 11.1 Sample High Blood Sugar Bolus Scale For A Hypothetical Pumper

If ketoacidosis is present or blood sugars have been high for some time, this person will need more bolus insulin than listed in the table above.

With experience, you will also discover when you need to take a bolus for high blood sugars occurring after meals. In certain circumstances, such as when a meal bolus was taken just before eating a food with a high glycemic index, a reading of 200 or 300 might be ignored because it will return to normal as the meal bolus takes effect. In many circumstances, however, blood sugars of 200 or 300 do not drop back to normal **unless extra insulin is taken**. It is important to understand what your own blood sugar will do and to have an individualized High Blood Sugar Bolus Scale to guide you in taking the correct bolus. Get guidance for this from your physician/health care team.

As an example, Table 11.1 shows a sample High Blood Sugar Bolus Scale for a person who weighs 160 pounds and has good control with an average of 38 units of insulin each day. The table was created after referring to Table 7.1 on page 50 to determine that this person's blood sugar was likely to drop about 40 points (rounded up from 37 mg/dl per unit of Reg.) for each unit of Regular. Target blood sugars were chosen as 100 mg/dl before a meal and 180 mg/dl two to three hours after a meal by this person and her physician. The scale gives the bolus insulin, in 0.5 unit increments, that the person will need for a high blood sugar that occurs before or after a meal.

Table 11.1 demonstrates what is called a sliding scale approach to lowering high blood sugars. **You would not use a High Blood Sugar Bolus, of course, if your blood sugars fall from high readings to normal on their own.**

TESTING HIGH BLOOD SUGAR BOLUSES

The High Blood Sugar Boluses in Table 7.1 are estimates that must be tested. Determine your own scale by testing and adjusting appropriately from the test results different from those estimated from Table 7.1. Table 11.2 on the next page shows how to test High Blood Sugar Boluses. You first select with help from your physician/health care team a Target Blood Sugar before meals (usually 90 to 140 mg/dl for testing purposes). You can do the test whenever a blood sugar above 180 mg/dl is found at least 5 hours after the last bolus of insulin was given, and at least 3 hours after the last food has been eaten. Eating must be delayed for another 5 hours to complete the test.

The ratio of Regular to the point drop in the blood sugar is tested and adjusted until the correct ratio is found that brings a high blood sugar to within 30 points of the selected target blood sugar 4 to 5 hours later. Test the blood sugar 2, 3, 4 and 5 hours after the test starts to reduce the risk of hypoglycemia. Repeat testing until a ratio is found that brings your blood sugar to normal on two consecutive tests. Then create your own personalized High Blood Sugar Bolus Scale as demonstrated in Table 11.1.

The High Blood Sugar Bolus Scale is one of the most important tools in helping you fine tune your blood sugar control. Combined with correct basal rates and meal boluses, the ability to lower high blood sugars safely is the last requirement for excellent control.

Caution: High Blood Sugar Boluses should be calculated in conjunction with the Unused Insulin Rule found in Chapter 12. Read that chapter before giving a High Blood Sugar Bolus. Remember also that your Target Blood Sugar is higher after meals than it is before meals.

Time	Action
Before The Test Begins	1. With your physician, select a Target Blood Sugar. Your Target Blood Sugar Value = _____ (usually 90 to 140 mg/dl for the test).
	2. Take no boluses for at least 5 hours before the test begins.
	3. Eat no food for at least 3 hours before the test begins.
	4. If conditions 2 & 3 are met, start the test whenever the blood sugar is over 200 mg/dl.
	5. Record your Starting Blood Sugar.
At The Start Of The Test	6. From Table 7.1, determine how far your blood sugar is likely to drop per unit of Regular.
	7. Subtract your Target Blood Sugar (Step 1) from your Starting Blood Sugar (Step 5). Difference (Step 1 minus Step 5) = _____.
	8. Divide the difference (Step 7) by the blood sugar drop per unit of Regular (Step 6). (Step 7) _____ ÷ (Step 6) _____ = _____ units of insulin.
	9. Take this bolus. DO NOT take it if it seems incorrect. Discuss first with your physician.
2, 3, And 4 Hours After The Start Of The Test	10. Test and record your blood sugar.
	a. If the blood sugar is 90 to 120 mg/dl at 2 or 3 hours, too much insulin may have been given. Test every 30 min.; if the blood sugar goes below 70, eat CHO & stop the test.
	b. If the blood sugar is higher than at the Starting Blood Sugar, check that your pump is working. Discuss whether to take more insulin with your physician/health care team.
5 Hours After The Start Of The Test	13. Test and record your blood sugar.
	a. If within 30 points of your Target Blood Sugar, the point drop per unit of Regular from Step 6 is correct. Retest to verify.
	b. If more than 30 points BELOW your target or you've had a low blood sugar, less insulin is needed. Try ADDING 5 points on the next test (i.e., if you used 1 unit/35 points this test, use 1 unit/40 points on the next test) to give yourself LESS insulin.
	c. If more than 30 points ABOVE your target, you may need more insulin. Check with your physician for advice about SUBTRACTING 5 points on the next test (if you used 1 unit/35 points this test, use 1 unit/30 points on the next test) to give yourself MORE insulin.

Table 11.2 How To Test How Far Your Blood Sugar Drops On A Unit Of Regular

If your blood sugar is low or likely to be low at any time, eat carbohydrate and stop the test.

Bolus Tips

- *Test Carbohydrate Boluses and High Blood Sugar Boluses **only after basal rates have been tested and accurately set**.*
- *Carbohydrate Boluses are determined by the carbohydrate in meals and snacks. Carbohydrate counting allows for optimum pump use.*
- *Carbohydrate Boluses: The correct ratio of Regular to grams of carbohydrate will return the blood sugar to within 30 points of the original blood sugar 5 hours after eating.*
- *High Blood Sugar Boluses: The correct ratio of Regular to number of points (mg/dl) the blood sugar will drop brings a high blood sugar to within 30 points of the Target Blood Sugar 5 hours after the bolus was given.*
- *Bolus insulin needs change when ketoacidosis, an infection, a change in weight, or a change in physical activity occur. Test more often when changing boluses for these reasons.*
- *If an unexpected high blood sugar occurs, the insulin pump should be immediately checked for leaks (O rings, hub, & catheter) and clogs (see Chapter 15).*
- *Signs of an incorrect ratio for the Carbohydrate Bolus:*
    *Too little insulin: when BG is OK before meals or snacks, but high BGs frequently occur after meals **and** before the next meal or at bedtime.*
    Too much insulin: when BG is OK before meals or snacks, but low BGs frequently occur after food is eaten.
- *Signs of an incorrect ratio for the High Blood Sugar Bolus:*
    Too little insulin: BG does not drop to Target as expected
    Too much insulin: BG frequently drops below Target
- If High Blood Sugar Boluses are required almost every day, either the basal rates or the Carbohydrate Boluses are too low.
- ***Quick Bolus Check:** Do boluses during the day make up 50 to 60% of the total daily insulin dose?*

"Too often we...enjoy the comfort of opinion without the discomfort of thought."

John F. Kennedy

The Unused Insulin Rule

12

One of the great advantages of an insulin pump is the ease of giving insulin. A bolus can be given for dinner, another bolus later for the unexpected dessert, then a high blood sugar bolus for the elevated reading two hours later. But a problem arises when insulin boluses start overlapping. How much insulin is still working? After several boluses, the bedtime blood sugar has to be interpreted in the light of **all the insulin that's still working**. A normal blood sugar at bedtime can be dangerous if one forgets the large residual dose of insulin that has yet to work. How much insulin or carbohydrate will you need once you've checked your bedtime blood sugar?

This chapter guides you through situations in which two or more boluses have been given over a period of 4 to 5 hours. This chapter:

- introduces the Unused Insulin Rule,
- shows how the Unused Insulin Table works, and
- points to discrepancies between the Unused Insulin Table and the High Blood Sugar Bolus Scale from Chapter 11 and ways to resolve them.

What Is The Unused Insulin Rule?

The Unused Insulin Rule tells you how many units of insulin are left working from previous boluses. This rule helps you decide whether you need more insulin or carbohydrate at any time of the day. Boluses from an insulin pump generally peak about 2 to 3 hours after they are given and most pumpers find that their blood sugars stop dropping from a bolus after 5 to 6 hours. This gives us the Unused Insulin Rule:

16% to 20% of an insulin bolus will be used each hour. From this rule, you can determine how much of a previous bolus has yet to work.

The 20%-an-hour guide works for those who are **more sensitive** to insulin. If you are younger and rarely take more than 10 units in a bolus, you will likely find little effect from your boluses 4 or 5 hours after the bolus is given. Insulin works longer in some people, however, and if you are older or take larger boluses, you may find your insulin is still lowering the blood sugar at 6 or 7 hours. If so, you will want to use the 16% guide.

How The Unused Insulin Rule Works

Tables 12.1 and 12.2 turn the Unused Insulin Rule into a practical tool. Table 12.1 (20% Rule) shows how much insulin is left from a previous bolus in those who get a **faster response** from their boluses and would normally be used by those who are younger and more physically active. Table 12.2 (16% Rule) on the next page shows how much insulin is left from a previous bolus in those who get a **slower response** from their insulin. Use the table that you feel is most appropriate for you to estimate how much insulin activity is left in the hours following one or more boluses.

Example 1: Let's say your blood sugar was off the scale of your meter (somewhere over 450 or 500 mg%) and you took a bolus 3 hours ago of 8 units to bring it down. You check your blood

Amount In Original Bolus	Units Of Regular Insulin Left After:				
	1 Hour	2 Hours	3 Hours	4 Hours	5 Hours
1 unit	0.8	0.6	0.4	0.2	0
2 units	1.6	1.2	0.8	0.4	0
3 units	2.4	1.8	1.2	0.6	0
4 units	3.2	2.4	1.6	0.8	0
5 units	4.0	3.0	2.0	1.0	0
6 units	4.8	3.6	2.4	1.2	0
7 units	5.6	4.2	2.8	1.4	0
8 units	6.4	4.8	3.2	1.6	0
9 units	7.2	5.4	3.6	1.8	0
10 units	8.0	6.0	4.0	2.0	0

Table 12.1 Faster Insulin Table (20%/hr): Use This Table Get a Quicker Action from Regular Insulin

sugar again and find it's now 300. Should you take additional insulin? To find out, let's use Table 12.1, assuming you are more sensitive to insulin. Using this table, you find that in 3 hours, 20% X 3 hours or 60% of your insulin activity is gone. You took 8 units, so 8 units X .60 = 4.8 units have been used. That means that 8 units - 4.8 units = **3.2 units are left**. (See Table 12.1 for confirmation.)

Let's say that your blood sugar drops 38 points on 1 unit of Regular. (See Table 7.1 to get a better estimate of your own blood sugar drop per unit of Regular.) You can then calculate the remaining activity of the earlier bolus as follows:

3.2 units left   X   38 points dropped per unit   =
121.6 points your blood sugar is still likely to drop from the previous bolus.

Since your blood sugar is 300, you can expect to be at 300 - 122 = 178 in another 2 hours when the remainder of the 8 unit bolus has been used. You now know you need to take more insulin if you want to lower your blood sugar to 100. You can then calculate how much more insulin to take:

178 - 100 = 78 more points to drop
78 points   ÷   38 points per units   =
2.0 more units needed to bring your blood sugar down.

Your calculations must be accurate to avoid an insulin reaction. Test frequently when using the Unused Insulin Rule. Do not use this much extra insulin at bedtime without your physician/health care team's advice. If they advise taking the extra insulin, set your alarm to wake up and test your blood sugar 2 or 3 hours after it was taken.

Amount In Original Bolus	Units Of Regular Insulin Left After:					
	1 Hour	2 Hours	3 Hours	4 Hours	5 Hours	6 Hours
1 unit	0.8	0.7	0.5	0.3	0.2	0
2 units	1.7	1.3	1.0	0.7	0.3	0
3 units	2.5	2.0	1.5	1.0	0.5	0
4 units	3.3	2.7	2.0	1.3	0.7	0
5 units	4.2	3.3	2.5	1.7	0.8	0
6 units	5.0	4.0	3.0	2.0	1.0	0
7 units	5.8	4.7	3.5	2.3	1.2	0
8 units	6.7	5.3	4.0	2.7	1.3	0
9 units	7.5	6.0	4.5	3.0	1.5	0
10 units	8.3	6.7	5.0	3.3	1.7	0

Table 12.2 Slower Insulin Table (16%/hr): Use This Table if You Get a Slower Action from Regular Insulin

Using the Unused Insulin Rule and how far your blood sugar drops on 1 unit of Regular, you are able to determine:

1. how much insulin is still active from previous boluses,

2. whether more insulin is needed to lower a high blood sugar **or** whether too much insulin has been taken, and

3. when more insulin is needed, how much is needed.

Example 2: As another example, let's say you go out for breakfast at a new restaurant. You order pancakes and fruit, but don't take your bolus until your food arrives because you're not sure how many carbohydrates it will have. When your plate arrives, you estimate you need 6.8 units aand take it. Two hours later your blood sugar is 193 mg/dl. You've previously found that your blood sugar drops 40 points on a unit of insulin. How much bolus do you need?

You took a bolus of 6.8 units and after 2 hours 40% of it has been used (20% X 2 hours). Since 60% of this bolus is still left:

$$6.8 \text{ units} \quad X \quad .60 \quad = \quad 4.1 \text{ units still active.}$$

Over the next 3 hours till the bolus is gone, your blood sugar will drop:

$$40 \text{ points dropped per unit} \quad X \quad 4.1 \text{ units left} \quad = \quad 164 \text{ more points to drop}$$

At that time your blood sugar will be:

$$193 \quad - \quad 164 \text{ points still to drop} \quad = \quad 29 \text{ (predicted blood sugar).}$$

It appears that not only is an additional bolus **not** necessary, but that **extra carbohydrate might be needed in the next hour or two**. A followup blood sugar in 60 to 90 minutes will clarify this. Eat extra carbohydrate at that time if needed.

RESOLVING DIFFERENCES BETWEEN THE UNUSED INSULIN RULE AND THE HIGH BLOOD SUGAR BOLUS SCALE

As you may have noticed in the last example, there are some discrepancies between how much insulin you estimate needing when you use two different methods: the Unused Insulin Rule described in this chapter and the High Blood Sugar Bolus Scale determined in Chapter 11.

If you had used the High Blood Sugar Bolus Scale in Example 2 when you had a blood sugar of 193 mg/dl 2 hours after eating, you would have calculated:

193 - 160 (your target blood sugar after eating) = 33 more points to drop
33 points to drop ÷ 40 points dropped per unit = 0.8 units of insulin still needed

By using your High Blood Sugar Bolus Scale, you would take a High Blood Sugar Bolus of 0.8 units of insulin. However, according to the Unused Insulin Rule **you really need more carbohydrate to prevent a low blood sugar.** Much of this discrepancy between the rules is due to having taken the bolus just before eating. You can't take a bolus just before eating and expect a post-meal reading of 160 mg/dl. This example points out that rules are never perfect. Rules provide guidance, but more important is basing your decisions upon your own judgement and experience, guided by the advice of your physician/health care team.

Tip: In the situation above, taking the breakfast bolus so close to the meal allowed the blood sugar to rise more than it would have otherwise. In this situation at a new restaurant, you can take a partial, safe bolus to lead the meal, and then catch up on the remainder of the meal bolus once you see the plate. Two hours is also a relatively short time to get a true reading of how well the meal bolus is going to cover that meal. A blood sugar at 3 hours after eating will be more precise.

The Unused Insulin Rule is more conservative than the High Blood Sugar Bolus Scale. That is, the Unused Insulin Rule is more likely to **overestimate** how much the blood sugar will drop and **underestimate** how much additional insulin may be needed. **It is intended to be conservative in order to avoid insulin reactions caused by chasing high blood sugars with too much insulin.**

Whenever there is a conflict between a bolus of insulin recommended by the Unused Insulin Rule and that recommended by your High Blood Sugar Bolus Scale:

1. consider first the bolus recommended by the Unused Insulin Rule,
2. then consider the bolus recommended by your High Blood Sugar BolusScale, and
3. decide on a bolus amount only after weighing all the factors that may affect your blood sugar. If in doubt, **always use the smaller bolus**.

Caution: When you have a high blood sugar and need to lower it with your pump, always check to be sure your pump has **really been giving you insulin**. Never take a bolus more often than every 2 or 3 hours. You need at least 3 hours to get an idea of what the last bolus is doing. Taking boluses more frequently allows too much insulin activity to build up, complicates your computations, and makes an insulin reaction likely.

"The only normal people are the ones you don't know very well."

Joe Ancis

PUMPING INSULIN

TREATING AND AVOIDING INSULIN REACTIONS

13

Insulin reactions are a major concern for most people using insulin. Mild reactions can be annoying and embarrassing, while a severe reaction can be dangerous. During a reaction, you may shake, sweat and feel disoriented. Or you may feel normal. A blood sugar of 60 or below will usually cause the release of excess stress hormones. Thinking and coordination often deteriorate as the blood sugar drops. Loss of coordination usually starts when the blood sugar goes below 60, although the loss may not be apparent to you. Regardless of how well you feel or think you feel, a blood sugar below 60 mg/dl is an insulin reaction and carries with it potential danger.

This chapter explores:

- some of the risk factors for reactions,
- symptoms of insulin reactions, both while awake and when asleep,
- key ways to avoid reactions,
- ways to treat reactions, and
- the special case of hypoglycemia unawareness.

WHAT CAUSES INSULIN REACTIONS?

Reactions are likely to happen:

- when too much insulin is being used (high basal, too much carbohydrate bolus, or too much high blood sugar bolus),
- when insulin is taken for a meal that is missed, delayed or interrupted,
- when large or frequent boluses are used to bring down high blood sugars,
- after drinking alcohol, and
- during or after exercise.

When beginning to use a pump, a person will often have difficulty accurately determining basal rates and boluses. This can be anticipated both because a pump has not been used before, and because using an insulin pump requires less insulin due to the physiologic delivery it provides. During this transition period, **insulin reactions are more likely**. **Keep in mind that insulin reactions themselves cause insulin reactions.** Researchers in Virginia found that a low blood sugar increases the risk of having another **low blood sugar**. They discovered that the chance of having a second insulin reaction following any reaction is greatly increased: 46% in the next 24 hours, 24% on the second day, 12% on the third day and only 2% on the fifth day after the original reaction.[70]

This extra vulnerability may also be increased by the natural enthusiasm, experimentation and uncertainty that accompanies the use of this new technology. Be aware of the pitfalls of your own enthusiasm and lack of experience with a pump. When first putting on a pump, most people are highly motivated. For the first time they have the technology for maintaining normal blood sugars. This feeling is positive and, in time, can lead to the goal of keeping blood sugars between 70 to 120 mg/dl before meals and no higher than 140 to 180 mg/dl after meals. Be willing, however, to set realistic goals, to pace yourself and to take small steps as you move toward a normal range.

Most importantly, be sure to check blood sugars often. Adjust basal and bolus insulins only with adequate testing. Adjust insulin doses gradually and in agreement with your physician/health care team's recommendation.

RECOGNIZING REACTIONS

Reactions can occur without symptoms, with minor symptoms, or with full blown symptoms. Symptoms vary from one person to another and from one reaction to another. Symptoms may first be recognized by the person having the reaction or by others. The type and degree of symptoms can vary depending on the speed and severity of the reaction. Recognizing insulin reaction symptoms is necessary to reduce risk.

New pumpers often find the symptoms they have during an insulin reaction are more subtle than when they were using injections. Pumps often lower the blood sugar more slowly than injections. This slower blood sugar drop actually gives the person more time to respond to a low blood sugar, but can also lower the blood sugar **with fewer symptoms**. This may require learning to respond to more subtle symptoms or different symptoms. Some common symptoms of insulin reactions are listed below.

SYMPTOMS FOR INSULIN REACTIONS

SWEATING
SHAKING
FAST HEART RATE
IRRITABILITY
SILLINESS
BLURRED VISION
DIZZINESS AND CONFUSION
FEELING TIRED SUDDENLY
HEADACHE
NAUSEA OR VOMITING
FREQUENT SIGHING
TINGLING
NUMBNESS OF THE LIPS

One or more of these symptoms can occur during any reaction; some may **never** occur. Check your blood sugar anytime an insulin reaction is suspected. Blood sugar testing will alert you to insulin reactions you may be having without symptoms.

FREQUENT OR SEVERE REACTIONS ALWAYS SUGGEST A CORRECTION IN INSULIN DOSES, CARBOHYDRATE INTAKE OR ACTIVITY IS NEEDED. MOST OFTEN, LESS INSULIN IS NEEDED.

RECOGNIZING NIGHTTIME REACTIONS

Symptoms for nighttime reactions can be particularly hard to recognize. Although reactions will be obvious when severe, more subtle symptoms can be hard to recognize, especially if someone awakens during the night in a reaction. It is also possible to sleep through a reaction and to have symptoms the next morning that are not recognized as caused by a reaction during the night. Below are symptoms that often occur during and after nighttime insulin reactions.

SYMPTOMS FOR NIGHTTIME REACTIONS

NIGHTMARES
WAKING UP WITH A FAST HEART RATE
DAMP NIGHT CLOTHES, SHEETS OR PILLOW
WAKING UP VERY ALERT DURING THE NIGHT
RESTLESSNESS AND INABILITY TO GO BACK TO SLEEP
UNUSUALLY HIGH BLOOD SUGAR AFTER BREAKFAST OR BEFORE LUNCH
A SMALL AMOUNT OF KETONES IN THE MORNING URINE
WAKING UP WITH A HEADACHE IN THE MORNING
LOSS OF MEMORY FOR WORDS OR NAMES
FEELING "FOGGY HEADED" ON WAKING

If you wake up during the night with any of the first five symptoms, check your blood sugar immediately. Eat quick-acting carbohydrates before checking if necessary. If you have any of the last five symptoms, you may have had an insulin reaction during the night. Review possible causes and take action to avoid a reoccurrence.

KEYS TO AVOIDING REACTIONS

- Test blood sugars often; use the results to control your blood sugars.
- Count your carbohydrates and match them with carbohydrate boluses.
- Eat the meals and snacks you take boluses for.
- Be careful when alcohol is involved; stupor and hypoglycemia have a lot in common.
- Test often before, during and after exercise.
- Be alert when changes in your daily routine are likely to affect your blood sugars.

TREATING INSULIN REACTIONS

Although prevention is the best treatment, not even the most conscientious person can prevent every reaction. When reactions occur, the best step is to relieve symptoms quickly. To prevent a high blood sugar following a low, do not **overtreat** the low blood sugar.

RELIEVE SYMPTOMS QUICKLY

For fast relief of symptoms, use glucose or dextrose. (Honey is also quite fast, but messy.) Glucose comes in tablets or tubes and can also be obtained in candies like Sweet Tarts®. Glucose is the "sugar" in "blood sugar." **Glucose tablets are made of dextrose, which consists of two glucose molecules.** Because dextrose is broken down quickly in the stomach to release 100% glucose into the blood, it is the best choice for raising blood sugars.

Table sugar is made from one glucose molecule and one fructose molecule. When table sugar breaks down in the stomach, **only 50% of it is immediately available as glucose**. Fruit juices, like orange juice, are made largely of fructose and are a poor choice for reactions because they take so long to raise the blood sugar.

Treating your insulin reactions with glucose tablets returns your blood sugar to normal more quickly than eating food. You feel better faster because brain, muscle and other cells receive the fuel they need faster. Raising the low blood sugar quicker also helps in shutting off the release of stress hormones and lowers the chance of having a high blood sugars after a reaction.

When raising blood sugars, a good rule of thumb is that 1 gram of glucose will raise the blood sugar 3 to 4 points. A 5 gram glucose tablet, for instance, should raise the blood sugar about 20 points. Sweet Tarts® come in different sizes. A popular one is the diameter of a Lifesaver roll but twice as long. Three Sweet Tarts® in this size roll equal 5 grams of carbohydrate, so for most reactions 6 to 9 tablets would be needed.

DON'T OVERTREAT

The second ingredient for success is moderation. **Don't go too far**. A panic overdose of orange juice with sugar, a box of chocolates or the entire contents of your refrigerator makes your goal of stable blood sugars hard to achieve. Panic reactions are caused by the release of stress hormones during lows. **It pays to be prepared for low blood sugars** by having glucose tablets, Sweet Tarts® or a pre-measured amount of quick carbohydrate handy. Some people find themselves gaining weight from overtreating reactions, which is another reason to avoid panicking.

One helpful way to decide how much carbohydrate is needed for a low blood sugar is to look at **how many hours have passed since the last bolus of insulin** was taken. If a bolus was taken only an hour or two ago, most of that last bolus has yet to act. More carbohydrate than normal will be needed. On the other hand, if the last bolus was 5 to 6 hours ago, a small amount of carbohydrate should easily correct the low.

THE BEST TREATMENT

The best treatment for reactions is a combination of simple and complex carbohydrates or protein. Ten to fifteen grams of simple carbohydrates, such as glucose tablets, Sweet Tarts® or honey, will quickly raise the blood sugar 40 to 60 points under most circumstances. Check to see how many grams of carbohydrate are in each glucose tablet you use.

Once you've eaten simple carbohydrates to raise your blood sugar quickly, have another 10 grams of complex carbohydrates, such as a small glass of milk or half an apple. Or eat high protein food, such as cheese or peanut butter or the glass of milk mentioned above. Both complex carbohydrates and proteins help keep the blood sugar from dropping later. Recheck your blood sugar a half hour after eating to be sure it has returned to normal. Of course, if you took a 10 unit bolus an hour ago in preparation for a meal and haven't eaten yet, a lot more carbohydrate than this will be needed.

Cognitive function, the ability to think, does not return to normal for 30 to 45 minutes after the blood sugar returns to normal. Avoid driving or operating machinery during this time.

1. Take 15 to 20 grams of quick-acting carbohydrates (glucose tablets, Sweet Tarts®, or honey).
2. Test your blood sugar 30 minutes later and treat it again if it is still low. Consider eating complex carbohydrates with protein (crackers and cheese or peanut butter, half an apple with cheese, or a cup of milk).
4. Wait 30 to 45 minutes after the blood sugar has returned to normal before driving or operating machinery.

Frequent or severe insulin reactions always indicate that too much insulin is being received. This is especially true if reactions:

- occur within 1 to 3 hours after a bolus, or
- require more than 15 grams of glucose to raise the blood sugar to normal.

If either of these situations is occurring, call your physician/health care team to discuss **an immediate decrease in your insulin**. If you tend to have low blood sugars, prevention of these reactions is always the best medicine. When an insulin pump is used well, a reduction in the number and severity of reactions should result. To insure that you're treating insulin reactions appropriately, chart what happens to your blood sugars **in the hours after you treat them**.

INSULIN REACTIONS AND DRIVING

Driving a car can at times be hypnotic or trancelike. With your attention on the road and other cars, you may not notice that your ability to think, to make decisions and to interact with others has changed. A slow drop in the blood sugar is especially hard to recognize while driving. As mentioned earlier, insulin reaction symptoms may be harder to notice on a pump. Don't drive if your blood sugar is below 70 mg/dl before starting the car or is likely to drop below 70 mg/dl at any time during the drive.

If you are driving a car and become involved in an auto accident due to a low blood sugar, many states will automatically suspend your license. **Always check your blood sugar before driving**. Make sure you have glucose tablets or Sweet Tarts® available. Some people always eat some carbohydrate prior to driving just to be safe. While driving, **stop** to test your blood sugar if you have any doubts. Don't be a statistic!

HYPOGLYCEMIA UNAWARENESS

New research is shedding light on one of the most distressing problems faced by a group of people who have diabetes (as well as their family, friends and co-workers). The problem, called hypoglycemia unawareness (HU), occurs when a person becomes incapable of dealing with his own low blood sugars. If unnoticed and untreated, HU can create serious problems, including grand mal seizures. If you've ever witnessed seizure activity or bizarre behavior in someone, you have some idea of the impact of HU and of its danger.

HU occurs when someone loses the ability to think during lows. They are unable to recognize that they are having a low blood sugar and cannot think clearly enough to correct it. A critical imbalance occurs in HU: thinking ability is lost **before** warning symptoms are severe enough for the person to recognize them. By the time the symptoms reach a serious level most people would recognize, the mind of the person with HU is not able to recognize the obvious shaking, nervousness and sweating. That this could occur during sleep is not surprising, but that it occurs while someone is awake is disturbing.

The risk of both hypoglycemia and HU increases as a person's average blood sugar is brought from high readings to normal. In the DCCT study, 55% of HU episodes occurred during sleep and they were three times as common in the intensively controlled group.

The mind normally recognizes reactions which allows a person to deal with the dropping blood sugar. But if the blood sugar drop is rapid, if someone has had diabetes for many years, if stress or depression are present, or if self-care is a low priority for any reason, the mind is less likely to recognize a reaction before it becomes truly severe. Reaction symptoms are less obvious after many years of diabetes because less epinephrine and glucagon are released. These stress hormones are needed to create the symptoms which make a reaction obvious.

Drinking alcohol is also a risk factor for HU. Alcohol contibutes to HU in three ways: the mind is less capable of recognizing what's happening, the liver is blocked from creating the glucose needed, and the release of free fatty acids (the backup to glucose for fuel) is also blocked.[71]

Researchers have discovered several ways to avoid HU. Keeping blood sugars slightly high, with better matching of insulin doses to diet and exercise is one way. Other options are keeping the warning signals active and keeping the brain cells operating under the duress of hypoglycemia.

A good way to lose one's warning signals is to recently have had a low blood sugar. Dr. Thiemo Veneman and other researchers demonstrated this principle in an article published in the November, 1993, issue of *Diabetes*.[72] Dr. Veneman and his group got 10 people who did NOT have diabetes to spend a day at the hospital on two occasions. While they slept, the researchers used insulin to lower their blood sugars to between 40 and 45 mg/dl for 2 hours in the middle of the night. (No, they didn't wake up! Most of us don't wake up during nighttime reactions. Memory serves us only for the reactions we wake up for.) Five people went through a nighttime low on the first visit and the other five on the second visit. Then, on waking in the morning, all were given insulin to lower their blood sugars to see when they would recognize they were getting low.

What Dr. Veneman found was that after sleeping through a reaction at night, people had **far more trouble** recognizing that their blood sugar was low the following day. Symptoms which warn us that a reaction is occurring come from the release of counter-regulatory hormones. These researchers found that stress hormones like epinephrine, norepinephrine and glucagon were released more slowly and in smaller concentrations after a nighttime reaction (actually after any reaction at all). In other words, a recent low makes it more likely that you'll fail to recognize a second low that follows the first.

In a major contribution to controlling HU, Dr. Carmine Fanelli and other researchers in Rome worked with people who had had their diabetes for seven years or less, but who suffered from HU.[73] The researchers and their subjects worked to reduce the frequency of insulin reactions by aiming for moderately higher premeal blood sugars (140 mg/dl). Frequency of hypoglycemia dropped from once every other day to once every 22 days. In raising premeal blood sugars, the researchers found that people who had previously had trouble recognizing their reactions were now able to do so. The counter-regulatory hormone response in these subjects returned to values that were nearly normal. These researchers demonstrated for the first time **that HU is reversible**.

Often other people can help someone who suffers from HU avoid a severe reaction if they recognize what is happening and take appropriate action. If someone with diabetes on insulin begins to act funny over a short period of time (usually 10 to 30 minutes), an insulin reaction is very likely and HU must be considered. A person's actions during HU can be bizarre with irrational thought, anger, irritability, running away, or insistence that he "feels fine" in the midst of behavior that is obviously unusual to others. Thinking is limited, fight or flight hormone levels are high, and an emotional reaction is likely. To help in this situation, gently coax and encourage the person with HU to eat or drink fast-acting carbohydrate. Demands upon and confrontation with an individual who already has high stress hormone levels is not wise.

Any plan to avoid HU will work only if the person who is having frequent lows or who has had HU in the past recognizes there is a problem to be dealt with. He or she must agree ahead of time to work with the spouse or co-workers in testing the blood sugar or eating if the support person requests this.

Obviously, keeping one's blood sugar target slightly higher, avoiding low blood sugars, and being especially careful following a first reaction are the best ways to prevent HU. The most important tool in treating HU is matching insulin to lifestyle. Someone who matches her insulin to changes in diet and life-style will be **less likely** to suffer from reactions and HU. For people with an active lifestyle, these insulin adjustments may need to be done daily. This is the appeal of multiple injections and insulin pumps: being able to adapt to the variability found in daily life, while encountering fewer and less severe insulin reactions.

Whenever insulin reactions are occurring frequently or whenever an episode of HU occurs, insulin doses must be lowered immediately. Discuss any situation like this with your physician that day. Avoiding frequent insulin reactions, including those occurring during the night, is also a very good policy in avoiding HU. An occasional 2 a.m. blood test can do wonders in preventing HU due to unrecognized nighttime reactions.

THE BEST WAYS TO PREVENT **HU**:

- KEEP THE BLOOD SUGAR TARGET SLIGHTLY HIGHER,
- AVOID LOW BLOOD SUGARS,
- *AND BE MORE CAREFUL IN THE HOURS THAT FOLLOW A FIRST REACTION.*

READING TEST FOR BRAIN DAMAGE:

*"People tell me one thing and out the other. I feel as much like I did yesterday as I did today.
I never liked room temperature. My throat is closer than it seems....
I don't like any of my loved ones."*

Daniel M. Wegner

PUMPING INSULIN

14

Exercise sharpens thought, calms the mind and tones the body. It increases self-esteem, energy and endurance, and provides a sense of well-being. It improves strength and efficiency in the heart and lungs, improves blood flow and oxygen availability, increases strength and elasticity of muscles, reduces body fat and weight, provides resistance against stress and fatigue, lowers triglyceride and LDL levels, and raises HDL levels.[74] **Lack of exercise** is itself a risk factor for heart disease, equivalent to smoking a pack of cigarettes a day or having high blood pressure or an elevated cholesterol level.

Exercise is especially important for the person with diabetes because of its specific benefit to the heart and blood vessels. Combining regular exercise and nutritious foods with the flexibility of insulin adjustments on an insulin pump helps keep blood sugars normal and stable. Good blood sugar control, in turn, further reduces risks for heart disease and other diabetes complications.

Exercise can improve blood sugar control. But if poorly planned and managed, it can easily cause loss of control. Why? Largely because of the demands exercise places on fuel flow. An increased need for fuel has to be met by a specific increase in the delivery of glucose and free fatty acids, or by reduction in insulin doses. The fuel used in exercise comes from foods, from internal stores of fat and glucose, and from glucose created by the liver. Accessing these fuels at the right time is complicated. A normal blood sugar during and after exercise means the demand for fuel and its supply are perfectly matched.

This chapter examines blood sugar control during exercise. In it we will:

- explain the importance of the insulin level during exercise,
- describe where fuel comes from, and
- provide guidelines for adjusting carbohydrates and insulin with exercise.

How Much Exercise?

A good first question is, how much exercise do I need? In a study of Harvard alumni, researchers found that lifespan increased steadily as people increased their exercise level from 500 calories to 3,500 calories per week.[75] The best results were reached when about 2,500 calories of energy were consumed each week by exercise. This is equivalent to walking 3 miles an hour for 7 hours a week, bicycling 10 miles an hour for 5 hours a week, or running 9 miles an hour for 2.7 hours a week. Increasing the intensity of exercise lessens the time required each week to obtain the same health benefit.

Erma Bombeck proclaimed, "The only reason I would take up jogging is so I could hear heavy breathing again." Fortunately in diabetes, exercise provides additional benefits beside that noted by Ms. Bombeck. Research conducted at the University of Wisconsin Medical School shows a marked lessening of eye damage in those who exercise.[76] The study ranked groups of people with Type I diabetes according to the amount of exercise they participated in, then looked at how much eye damage they had. The researchers found that proliferative diabetic retinopathy occurred in 36% of sedentary women but in only 16% of those who were very physically active. In men, severe eye damage dropped from 48% in sedentary men to 16% in those very physically active.

Intensity may not be as important in the prevention of heart disease as it is in the prevention of retinopathy. Regular moderate exercise has been noted to have as much benefit in protecting the heart as strenuous exercise. If burning 2,500 calories each week is too much, try moderate exercise. Brisk walking or bicycling for 30 minutes 5 days a week, helps prevent heart disease.[75] Using 1,000 calories per week in exercise appears to have major benefits to health. This is especially good news to many people who find brisk walking more appealing than running marathons.

The International Diabetic Athletes Association (1931 E. Rovey Ave.; Phoenix, Arizona 85016; [602] 230-8155) holds a three-day North American Conference each year with talks and workshops on many different sports. One finding presented by several exercise specialists at the August, 1993 conference, and confirmed by participants, is that the more muscle mass one has, the easier blood sugar control becomes. This suggests that a combination of **aerobic exercise** for cardiovascular fitness and **strength training** for muscle mass is important in diabetes.

CAUTIONS ABOUT EXERCISE

Although exercise is generally very positive to health, some cautions are needed. Be sure to discuss your exercise plans with your physician/health care team before starting, especially if you have any diabetes-related damage, such as nerve damage, eye changes, kidney disease, or a history of heart or blood vessel problems. Exercise increases blood flow and blood pressure as oxygen and fuels are pumped to exercising muscles. Blood flow to muscles may increase 15-fold to 20-fold during strenuous exercises. This can harm organs and blood vessels weakened by past high blood sugars. This has to be considered **before beginning an exercise program**.

The presence of nerve damage also presents some challenges. If feeling has been lost in the feet, normal position and pain sensations are not received. Damage may occur if exercise stresses the feet, but the lack of foot pain prevents the athlete from being aware of this damage. This does not mean exercise should not be done. Rather, consideration has to be given to the type of exercise and to adequate protection of the feet.

Pumpers vary greatly in how their blood sugars respond to exercise. Some require large amounts of additional carbohydrate for exercise, some none. The same pumper may require different amounts of carbohydrate for the same amount of exercise done at different times of the day or on different days. Therefore, discuss your exercise program with your physician/health care team, monitor your blood sugars often, and use the information on exercise provided in this book.

DOES BLOOD SUGAR LEVEL AFFECT PERFORMANCE?

The blood sugar of a nondiabetic athlete usually stays between 70 and 85 mg/dl during even the most strenuous exercise. Precise blood sugar control is important for performance. Athletes who have diabetes report that performance is highest when blood sugars are as normal as possible, especially between 70 and 150 mg/dl. Why this range is important becomes apparent when considering what happens beyond it, as outlined in Table 14.1.

Muscle efficiency depends on the blood sugar, so testing opens the door to maximum athletic performance. A normal blood sugar during exercise allows maximum energy output. It also allows the muscles and heart to receive glucose and fat in amounts that allow them to function well.

Blood Sugar Level	Effect of Sugar Level on Metabolism	Effect of Sugar Level on Performance
<65	Too little sugar is in the blood to fuel muscle or brain cells.	Tiredness and poor performance.
65-150	Efficient fuel flow.	Maximum Performance
>150	Sugar has trouble entering muscle cells,* esp. with low insulin levels.	Mildly reduced performance.
>250	With moderate or strenuous exercise and low insulin levels, blood sugars can rapidly rise.	Tiredness and poor performance.**

Table 14.1 Effect of Blood Sugar on Metabolism and Performance.

* Exception to this occurs if a bolus had been given and insulin levels are on the rise (despite the temporary high blood sugar), or if the insulin deficit is small and prolonged exercise is planned.

** Bring the blood sugar below 250 before exercising. Determine why the blood sugar is high and recheck every 1 to 2 hours until control is regained.

WHAT'S INVOLVED IN BALANCING BLOOD SUGARS WITH EXERCISE?

When traveling by car, you can easily determine how much gasoline is needed for a trip. Once you know how long the trip will take (duration), the speed at which you'll drive (intensity), and the miles per gallon your car gets at that speed, you can calculate the number of gallons of gasoline (energy) needed. Mileage is determined by a car's weight and by engine efficiency. Control of gasoline is determined by a properly adjusted carburetor. The number of gallons of gas used in the trip equals the amount of energy expended. If you put this amount of gasoline back into your gas tank, you can repeat the trip.

Exercise is similar in some ways to a car trip. If someone weighs 150 pounds and runs 30 minutes (duration) at 7 m.p.h. (intensity or speed), he or she can determine the amount of energy, about 320 calories in this case, used in the run. But the human body is more flexible than a car in two important ways:

- the insulin level or "human carburetor" is not precisely set, but adjusts to meet the intensity and duration of various forms of exercise, and
- the body can use two fuels, glucose and fat, rather than a car's single fuel, gasoline.

Muscle performance depends on the release of glucose and fat as fuel, with over 90% of the energy needed for exercise derived from these sources. Glucose in the blood and glycogen stores in muscle and liver are tapped first, but these supplies are limited. During strenuous exercise, sugar in the blood is used in about 4 minutes compared to 30 minutes at rest.[77] Glycogen reserves available from the liver are sent into the bloodstream and depleted in another 20 minutes.

The "wall" often encountered by marathon runners at 20 to 24 miles into the race results from the depletion of glucose and glycogen resources by this demanding exercise. To enlarge their glycogen stores, athletes often carbohydrate-load before major events by eating large amounts of complex carbohydrates. Then over an 8 to 30 hour period following a major exercise event, glucose is removed from the blood into muscle glycogen to replenish these stores.

Free fatty acids are mobilized from the large stores of energy in fat cells. Free fatty acids are better mobilized from these stores if insulin levels in the blood are lowered during exercise.

Why Is The Insulin Level Important?

The insulin level helps to regulate which fuel is used in exercise. Too much insulin in the blood will cause problems as will too little. For the nondiabetic, these problems are avoided by **rapid changes in blood insulin levels**. At the start of **strenuous** exercise, the blood insulin level begins to drop, reaching 50% of the pre-exercise level **in about 15 minutes**.[78] With moderate exercise, about an hour passes before a similar drop in the blood insulin level is seen.

Lowering the blood insulin level at the start of exercise allows the body to change its fuel source. Instead of being able to only use the sugar in the blood, a lower insulin level lets glucose be mobilized out of glycogen stores in the muscles and liver, new glucose be created in the liver, and free fatty acids be mobilized from fat cells. The blood sugar remains steady as glucose used in exercise is replenished from these large glucose stores, and as more energy is obtained from very large stores of fat. This prevents blood sugar levels from dropping as sugar is shifted into exercising muscles.

> ### Chromium & Vanadium
>
> The trace minerals chromium and vanadium enhance the glycogen supply inside muscle cells, especially when combined with exercise. Chromium helps insulin attach to cell membranes. It reportedly helps to stabilize blood sugar levels, possibly by enhancing the glycogen buffering system inside these cells. Exercise also helps to stabilize control by this buffering mechanism. In research studies, vanadium, in very large doses, has insulin-like effects and reduces appetite. It rapidly normalizes blood sugars in mice with Type I diabetes. **Unfortunately, at the doses required, many of the mice died from the vanadium treatment.** Whether doses of vanadium useful for humans can be found hasn't been determined. Chromium picolinate at levels of 50 to 200 mcg. a day appears to be safe and useful.

A precise, rapid adjustment in insulin level allows someone without diabetes to exercise and do strenuous work for prolonged periods without eating. But in diabetes, insulin levels are not automatically adjusted. Thought and care have to be given to set insulin levels correctly. If insulin levels are **too high**, sugar in the blood will enter exercising muscles quickly while a person is unable to release stores from glycogen. This causes a falling blood sugar and finally an insulin reaction, unless the blood sugar was high when the exercise began or carbohydrate is eaten.

On the other hand, when blood insulin levels are **too low**, sugar has trouble getting into exercising muscles, but stored glucose and free fatty acids are being easily moved into the blood. This causes blood sugars to rise during exercise. Table 14.2 shows some of the effects the insulin level has on blood sugar levels, stress hormone levels, and glucose and free fatty acid metabolism.

Although the insulin level directly affects performance, **it's not easy to measure**. A low blood sugar always indicates excess insulin. But high blood sugars have to be judged in context. The advice that's generally given is: don't exercise if your blood sugar is over 250 mg/dl. Although usually sound advice, it's not always true.

When a high blood sugar occurs first thing in the morning, it shows a lack of insulin. Exercising at this time is likely to raise the blood sugar even higher. But in preparing for an athletic event, some athletes with diabetes will reduce their insulin dose and eat extra carbohydrate.

Insulin Level:	Effect on Stress Hormones	Effect on Glucose and Fat	Effect on Blood Sugar
Low	Excess release of stress hormones	Glucose is less able to enter exercising muscle. Glucose release, glucose production and free fatty acid release are all increased.	A high blood sugar. Possible ketosis.
Ideal	Normal release of stress hormones	Glucose entry into exercising muscle is appropriate. Supplies of glucose and free fatty acids are released in the correct amounts.	A normal blood sugar. Optimum performance.
High	Decreased release of stress hormones	Glucose is more able to enter cells. Release of both glucose and free fatty acids is blocked.	A low blood sugar. Poor performance.

Table 14.2 How The Blood Insulin Level Affects Stress Hormones, Glucose, Free Fatty Acids and Blood Sugars During Exercise.

Although they may start the event with a blood sugar that has rapidly risen to 200 or 300 mg/dl, the sugar will quickly drop shortly into the event because they have enough insulin to move the glucose into exercising muscles.

On the pump, of course, an alternative is to **lower** the basal insulin a couple of hours before the event and eat less carbohydrate before and during the event. Because the insulin level is lowered and less carbohydrate has to be eaten, a high blood sugar is avoided and there is **less risk of an insulin reaction**.

As another example of the importance of the insulin level, during **very strenuous exercise** glucose is rapidly released into the blood, driven by rising stress hormone levels. This newly released glucose must be moved into exercising muscle to prevent the blood sugar from rising. To do this, the nondiabetic will quickly **double the amount of insulin in the blood**. The athlete with diabetes cannot do this and may instead see a rapid rise in the blood sugar level after very strenuous events, even though he or she starts with a normal blood sugar. Instead of lower insulin doses recommended for most exercise, a small bolus of Regular may be needed prior to **very strenuous** exercise to prevent high blood sugars. Never give a bolus before strenuous exercise without first discussing it with your physician/health care team, and only after extensive testing has demonstrated that this insulin is needed.

Everyone must adapt to the way his or her own blood sugars respond to exercise. To learn how to change your insulin doses for different types of exercise, you have to experiment. Follow the suggestions in Table 14.6 for adjusting your basal rates, boluses, and carbohydrate intake. Then test your blood sugar before, during and after exercise. Feedback gained through such trial and error will let you adjust your insulin doses for the length and intensity of your own exercise. Always keep fast-acting carbohydrate easily available for lows.

WHAT'S THE IMPACT OF THE INTENSITY AND DURATION OF EXERCISE?

When a person is at rest, most fuel is supplied by free fatty acids. In mild exercise, like walking or golfing, energy is still largely obtained from fats rather than sugar. For this reason, a drop in the blood sugar is less likely during mild exercise. **As exercise intensity increases, so does the use of sugar for fuel.** Walking or running a mile makes no difference in the amount of energy used. Moving yourself the same distance at any speed uses almost the same number of calories. But in a one-mile walk, only 20% of the calories may come from sugar, whereas as much as 80% of calories may come from sugar during a strenuous mile run. Fat makes up the difference.

Because of the greater use of carbohydrate during intense exercise, exercise that is strenuous is more likely to cause a blood sugar drop. **Strenuous exercise, therefore, has to be balanced with more carbohydrate intake or a larger reduction in insulin than milder types of exercise** (with the exception of *very strenuous* exercise noted above).

How long exercise lasts also influences how much carbohydrate is used. **Activities that last longer drop the blood sugar more.** For instance, a 30-minute walk might not affect the blood sugar, but walking for 60 minutes may require extra carbohydrate or a lower meal bolus. With experience, your ability to estimate the intensity and length of upcoming activities improves, along with your ability to balance them with extra carbohydrate or less insulin. Tables 14.3 and 14.4 show how duration and intensity affect whether the body needs carbohydrate or fat as fuel. To keep blood sugar levels normal, fuel used in exercise has to be eaten as carbohydrate, released from internal stores, or created by the liver.

How Long?	Fuel Preferred
Short	Glucose
Medium	Glucose & Fat
Long	Fat

Table 14.3 How Duration Affects The Fuel Used

How Hard?	Fuel Preferred
Mild	Fat
Moderate	Fat & Glucose
Vigorous	Glucose & Fat
Strenuous	Glucose

Table 14.4 How Intensity Affects The Fuel Used

As exercise intensity increases, more calories are used per hour and a **higher percentage** of these calories has to be obtained from glucose. But as exercise continues, the body begins to switch from using its limited stores of glucose and glycogen for energy to using the very large stores of fat in the body. Figure 14.1 shows the normal person's body shifting to use more fat as exercise continues over several hours. In this example, the person is getting 80% of his or her energy from glucose at the start of fairly strenuous exercise. At 3 hours he or she is using equal amounts of glucose and fat, but at the end of 6 hours almost 80% of the energy is being derived from fat. Remember, though, this person has a normal pan-

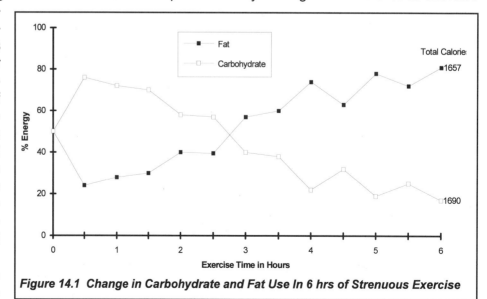

Figure 14.1 Change in Carbohydrate and Fat Use In 6 hrs of Strenuous Exercise

creas that **automatically lowers insulin levels**. If someone with diabetes does not reduce his or her insulin doses for this same exercise, he or she will be less able to access fat for fuel and be **forced to eat carbohydrate** to supply this energy.

The numbers to the right of the carbohydrate and fat lines show the total amount of energy in calories that come from each source. The total energy used was 3,347 calories, with 1,690 calories coming from carbohydrate and 1,657 calories from fat. If someone with diabetes **kept his or her insulin level high** during this 6 hours of exercise, the excess insulin would block access to both fat and glycogen stores in the body. With internal stores largely blocked, to keep blood sugars from falling **3,347 calories of carbohydrate would have to be eaten**. This means eating almost two pounds of pure sugar, or drinking 20 twelve ounce cans of regular soda. Obviously, lowering insulin levels helps prevent both low blood sugars and stomach aches.

DOES YOUR LEVEL OF TRAINING MAKE A DIFFERENCE?

Because they are less efficient, **untrained muscles use more glucose for the same amount of exercise**. Someone who is poorly trained uses **about 25% more glucose** for the same exercise as someone well-trained. Each muscle cell has its own internal supply of sugar called glycogen. As untrained muscles exercise, they pull in more sugar from the bloodstream than trained muscle cells because untrained cells have smaller internal stores of glycogen.

Following the start of a new type of exercise, **extra carbohydrate** is needed by untrained muscles due to less efficient use of glucose, and to a buildup of glycogen stores following the exercise. This post-exercise glycogen buildup occurs over several hours after any new exercise, as muscle cells resupply and enlarge glycogen stores in preparation for more of this exercise in the future. This buildup causes a delayed drop in blood sugar **after the exercise**, often during sleep that night. A nighttime reaction often happens when starting a new exercise program or when resuming an activity not recently participated in. As training improves over time, glycogen stores enlarge, muscle efficiency increases, and blood sugars become less likely to drop.

A post-exercise drop also occurs when exercise involves different muscle groups, for example, in running versus biking. A runner who begins to bike will have a larger blood sugar drop after biking than after running, even though the length and intensity of the exercise are the same.

Extra carbohydrate should always be handy for exercise, especially following random, intense exercise for which one has not trained. Examples of this are canoe trips, backpacking, skiing, horse riding, spring cleaning, home remodeling, or hoeing and shoveling in the garden.

Another way for someone who is poorly trained to offset exercise safely is to **lower the insulin level**. This helps the body access fat for fuel during and after exercise. As insulin doses are lowered, however, blood sugars should continue to remain normal. A normal blood sugar indicates that an ideal balance has been reached for using both glucose and fat as fuels.

To Summarize:

**The longer the exercise period,
the more intense the exercise,
the less trained the muscles, or
the higher the insulin level,**

the more likely the blood sugar is to drop!

CARBOHYDRATE ADJUSTMENTS

Eating carbohydrate is a rapid and convenient way to balance most exercise. The energy needed to exercise is provided by eating the grams of carbohydrate the exercise consumes. No meal bolus is taken to cover this free carbohydrate. It can be eaten before, during and after exercise based on blood sugar test results.

The calories used in a particular exercise are easy to determine from standard tables. From a person's weight and fitness level and from the duration and intensity of exercise, a good estimate of calorie replacement can be made for a particular exercise. For example, someone who weighs 150 pounds and runs 7 miles an hour (intensity) for 30 minutes (duration) will consume about 320 calories of energy. Most of these calories need to be replaced by carbohydrate, with each gram of carbohydrate equal to 4 calories.

Table 14.5 on the next page gives the grams of carbohydrate needed to replace one hour of some common exercises. These estimates are **generous** to provide a margin for error. Less carbohydrate than shown may actually be needed, except when insulin levels are excessive or training is poor. If you regularly need more than these generous amounts of carbohydrate for a type of exercise or you have frequent insulin reactions due to exercise, you will want to look at lowering your insulin doses. Talk with your physician/health care team for guidance on doing this.

Table 14.5 assumes that

- you are well trained for the exercise,
- basals and boluses are correctly set when you're not exercising,
- if a meal bolus is to be lowered before an exercise that lasts more than 45 or 60 minutes, **less** carbohydrate will be needed (see Table 14.6), and
- if basal rates are lowered for exercise that lasts more than 60 minutes, **less** carbohydrate will be needed (see Table 14.6).

Table 14.5 gives the expected carbohydrate needed for one hour of these types of exercise by people who weigh 100, 150, or 200 pounds. Adjustments will need to be made for your own weight. For example, if a person weighs 170 pounds and plans to walk 3 miles in an hour, he or she should need a maximum of 32 grams of carbohydrate for this walk. Again: **no insulin** is taken to cover the carbohydrate eaten for the walk.

Different carbohydrates raise the blood sugar at different speeds and can be chosen to accomplish different goals. Fast carbs are ideal for raising low blood sugars before or during exercise, and also when exercise consumes carbohydrate rapidly. Slower carbs are great for preventing lows during long periods of activity. Slow carbs work best when eaten at least 30 minutes before exercise begins, and at about 45 minute intervals thereafter.

Fast Carbs: glucose tablets, Sweet Tarts, honey, Cornflakes, Raisin Bran, athletic drinks (Exceed, Body Fuel), raisins, dried fruit, regular soft drinks, apple juice.

Slow Carbs: athletic bars (PowerBar, PurePower), oatmeal, Swiss muesli, Cheerios, fruit, Fig Newtons, Teddy Grahams, ginger snaps, pasta, brown rice, candy bars (high fat).

Activity/Exercise	Weight			Activity/Exercise	Weight		
	100 lbs	150 lbs	200 lbs		100 lbs	150 lbs	200 lbs
Walking at 3 mi/hr	14	21	28	Raking Leaves/Hoeing	20	30	40
Jogging at 5 mi/hr	30	45	60	Ice Skating/Roller Skating	23	34	45
Running at 7 mi/hr	52	77	103	Trampoline	23	35	47
Running at 9 mi/hr	69	103	138	Digging a Garden	23	35	47
Bicycling at 5 mi/hr	13	20	27	Ice Skating at 10 mi/hr	23	35	47
Bicycling at 10 mi/hr	30	45	60	Chopping Wood	23	35	47
Bicycling at 15 mi/hr	52	77	103	Disco Dancing	24	36	48
Swimming at 20 yds/min	24	36	48	Hand Mower	25	38	51
Light Gardening	8	12	16	Single Tennis	25	38	51
Golfing with Golfcart	9	14	19	Square Dancing (Fast)	29	44	59
Mopping Floors	12	18	24	Waterskiing	29	44	59
Power Lawn Mower (Push)	13	19	25	Snow Shovelling	30	45	60
Bowling	13	19	25	Digging Ditches	31	46	62
Golfing with Pullcart	13	20	27	Rock Climbing	31	46	62
Scrubbing Floors	17	25	33	Dancing (Fast Step)	31	46	62
Softball	17	25	33	Downhill Skiing	33	50	67
Badminton	19	28	37	Pickup Basketball	39	58	77
Horseback Riding (Trot)	19	28	37	Squash	40	60	80
Square Dancing (Slow)	19	28	37	Soccer	40	60	80
Doubles Tennis	19	28	37	Basketball (Vigorous)	44	65	87
Roller Skating	21	31	42	Singles Racquetball	60	90	120
Volleyball	21	31	42	Crosscountry Skiing, 6 mph	70	105	140

Table 14.5 Average Grams Of Carbohydrate Needed For Each Hour Of Various Exercises

Carb Contents: Body Fuel: 10 grams/8 oz.   Exceed Fluid: 17 grams/8 oz.
                      apple juice: 27 grams/8 oz.   orange juice: 25 grams/8 oz.
                      regular soda: 40 grams/12 oz.   Gatorade: 12 grams/8 oz.

                      PowerBar: 40 grams carb, 2 grams fat, 10 grams protein
                      PurePower: 42 grams carb, 3 grams fat, 12 grams protein
                      Exceed Bar: 53 grams carb, 2 grams fat, 12 grams protein
                      Snickers: 36 grams carb, 13 grams fat, 5 grams protein

INSULIN ADJUSTMENTS

Insulin always lowers the blood sugar; exercise usually does. If exercise is short and mild, the best way to balance it is to simply eat extra carbohydrate. As exercise increases in length and intensity, a reduction in insulin doses becomes more and more necessary. Long, intense periods of exercise **require** that insulin levels be lowered before the exercise starts, and that they be kept lower for several hours following the exercise. Eating extra carbohydrate will also be required.

With the ease of insulin dose adjustments on a pump, the rapid changes in blood insulin levels required for longer or strenuous periods of exercise become easier to make. This is done by lowering boluses for meals just before exercise begins and/or lowering the basal rate. Smaller meal boluses are ideal for moderate or strenuous exercise that occurs within 2 hours of eating.

When the basal rate is lowered, it takes **90 to 120 minutes** to start lowering the insulin level in the blood. So lowering the basal rate has to be planned in advance. (The temporary basal rate feature on some pumps is very handy for this.) Lowering the basal rate is ideal for moderate or strenuous exercise that lasts 60 minutes or longer and may be required to prevent low blood sugars after exercise has stopped. Table 14.6 gives suggested reductions in basal rates and boluses for the length and intensity of exercise.

Unlike carbohydrates which can be added as needed, **insulin doses can be reduced only so far**. How far boluses and basals can be lowered is determined by:

- the need to cover meal carbohydrates with enough insulin to prevent the blood sugar from rising too high after the meal, and
- the need for enough background insulin to allow glucose entry into cells and to prevent an excessive release of glucose and fat from internal stores.

Even with the most intense forms of exercise, such as running a marathon or competing in a triathelon, **the total daily insulin dose cannot be reduced more than 40% to 50%.** Some tips for adjusting insulin:

- For exercise lasting less than an hour and occurring within 3 hours of a meal, you can:
    1. eat extra carbohydrate and not lower the bolus for the meal,
    2. lower the normal meal bolus by 30% to 50%, or
    3. reduce the meal bolus by 20% and eat extra carbohydrate.
- The basal rate rarely needs to be lowered for short, random periods of exercise, but may need to be lowered if exercise is done frequently to increase physical fitness.
- For intense activities that last a day or two, such as a weekend backpacking trip, try lowering the basal rate by 20% to 40% and boluses by 50%. Lower the basal rate 2 hours before the activity begins and continue it for as long as 24 hours after it has ended.

- When beginning a period of **vigorous** training, lower the basal rate substantially. For instance, if the basal rate has been correctly set before beginning a vigorous training program, a reduction in the basal rate of 20% to 40% is often needed.
- The normal Carbohydrate Bolus may need to be lowered by 50% or more when taken before or during vigorous exercise or heavy work. For example, if 1 unit is normally taken for each 10 grams of carbohydrate, try taking only 1 unit for every 18 or 20 grams when working or exercising hard. Some vigorous exercise may require the total elimination of a meal bolus.
- The normal High Blood Sugar Bolus may need to be reduced by 40% to 70% when given before or during periods of vigorous exercise.

COMBINED INSULIN AND CARBOHYDRATE ADJUSTMENTS

Table 14.6 gives recommendations about how to adjust carbohydrates, basal rates and boluses to match exercise with various durations and intensities. **Adjustments of insulin and carbohydrate vary greatly from individual to individual.** Some people may lower the basal rate or boluses for exercise only slightly; others may find that a large insulin reduction is the only way to control blood sugars while exercising. The only way to determine this is to **cautiously experiment** and **discuss your results with your physician/health care team**. Test your blood sugar often while experimenting. The reasons for these variations from one person to the next are complex and not completely understood.

Refer back to Table 14.5 for the number of grams of carbohydrate needed to offset a particular exercise when no adjustment of basal rates or boluses is planned. Once you have determined the number of grams of carbohydrate needed for your exercise, you can choose to offset that amount of carbohydrate by:

- eating that number of grams of carbohydrate,
- reducing meal boluses,

Duration	Intensity								
	Mild			**Moderate**			**Intense**		
	CHO	Bolus	Basal	CHO	Bolus	Basal	CHO	Bolus	Basal
15 min.	No Adj.	No Adj.	No Adj.	No Adj.	No Adj.	No Adj.	▲	No Adj.	No Adj.
30 min.	No Adj.	No Adj.	No Adj.	▲	No Adj.	No Adj.	▲	▼	No Adj.
45 min	▲	No Adj.	No Adj.	▲	▼	No Adj.	▲	▼▼	No Adj.
60 min	▲	▼	No Adj.	▲	▼	No Adj.	▲▲	▼▼	▼
120 min	▲	▼	No Adj.	▲▲	▼▼	▼	▲▲	▼▼▼	▼▼
240 min	▲▲	▼	No Adj.	▲▲	▼▼▼	▼	▲▲▲	▼▼▼	▼▼

Bolus: ▼ = 30% lower   ▼▼ = 50% lower

Basal: ▼ = 20% lower   ▼▼ = 40% lower

Table 14.6 Suggested Insulin Adjustments for Various Intensities and Durations of Exercise

- reducing basal rates,
- allowing the exercise to drop a high blood sugar, or
- some combination of the above.

Eating an equal amount of carbohydrate is easy for exercise that is less than an hour in length and mild or moderate in intensity. As length and intensity of exercise increase, so does the quantity of food required to offset the exercise. At some point, a reduction in insulin doses becomes necessary.

Let's say you weigh 200 pounds, use 45 units a day with your pump and have excellent control. From Table 7.1 on page 50 you'll need 1 Regular for each 10 grams of carbohydrate and 1 Regular for each 33 points you wish to lower your blood sugar. You wake up one morning with a blood sugar of 166 and plan to eat a breakfast containing 100 grams of carbohydrate, then ride a bike 15 miles in an hour (intense exercise for you). Usually you would take 10 units for breakfast and 2 units for the high blood sugar. You calculate from Table 14.5 that at 200 pounds and riding a bike at 15 m.p.h., you'll use the equivalent of 103 grams of carbohydrate for the ride. This 103 grams can be translated into:

- 10.3 fewer units of insulin (103/10 grams per unit),
- a blood sugar drop of 340 points (33 point drop per unit X 10.3 units), or
- an extra 103 grams of free carbohydrate.

So your choices become:

1. Take 12 units of insulin---10 units for the breakfast carbohydrate, plus 2 extra units for the high blood sugar. Then eat 100 grams of carbohydrate for breakfast, plus another 103 grams of free carbohydrate during and after the bicycle ride. This extra 103 grams of carbohydrate equals **seven** average slices of bread.

2. Or take 2 units to lower the blood sugar, but only 5 units to cover breakfast (the usual breakfast bolus cut in half); then eat your planned 100 gram carbohydrate breakfast. The lower insulin level allows better access to internal glucose stores. A smaller amount of extra carbohydrate (20 to 50 grams) will then be needed during and after the ride.

INSULIN REACTIONS AND EXERCISE

A low blood sugar during exercise or strenuous work is often difficult to sense. Symptoms like sweating and shaking may be due to the exercise or work, or may be due to a low blood sugar. Normal warning signals may go unnoticed due to involvement in an activity. Monitoring regularly during exercise prevents reactions, as well as allowing better performance.

LOWS DURING EXERCISE

Low blood sugars that occur during and immediately after exercise are caused by not eating enough carbohydrate for that exercise or from exercising while having a blood insulin level that is too high. When someone exercises with a high blood insulin level, an insulin reaction can occur even if the blood sugar was high at the start of exercise. For example, if someone takes a large bolus to cover carbohydrate intake just before exercise begins, the resulting high blood insulin level will block the release of glucose from glycogen stores and the release of free fatty acids from fat stores. The result can be a rapid drop in the blood sugar.

Lows After Exercise

Delayed reactions frequently follow strenuous or prolonged exercise or work. **They can occur up to 36 hours later and frequently happen in the middle of the night.** Delayed reactions are caused by the gradual drop in blood sugars as muscle cells remove sugar from the blood to replenish their glycogen stores depleted during exercise. Delayed reactions following strenuous exercise can be prevented by testing blood sugars more often, by lowering basal rates for the next 36 hours and by eating more carbohydrate, especially at bedtime.

Remember: Exercise easily masks the symptoms of a low blood sugar.

Exercise Tips

- Most exercise requires extra carbohydrate and/or lowered insulin doses to prevent low blood sugars.
- Lowering boluses and basal rates allows access to internal stores of glucose and fat during prolonged exercise. Lowering insulin also helps prevent low blood sugars during and after exercise.
- For performance and safety, the blood sugar should be between 70 and 150 mg/dl while exercising. After exercise it should not drop below 65 mg/dl.
- Eating carbohydrate is a rapid, convenient way to balance exercise. Body weight and the intensity and duration of the exercise determines the amount of carbohydrate needed (see Tables 14.4 and 14.5).
- The longer and more strenuous the exercise is, the more likely a blood sugar is, and the more likely it is that insulin has to be lowered (see Table 14.5).
- The less training one has for an exercise, the more likely the blood sugar is to drop.
- *Very strenuous* exercise can raise the blood sugar if glucose is mobilized faster than it can be moved into cells by the prevailing insulin level.
- Extra blood sugar testing is needed before and after exercise, during exercise that lasts over 45 minutes, and whenever low blood sugar symptoms occur. If exercise is intense or lengthy, monitor frequently over the next 24 to 36 hours.
- For rapid correction of low blood sugars during exercise, carry fast-acting carbohydrates, like glucose tablets or SweetTarts®.

"I don't jog. If I die, I want to be sick."

Abe Lemons

PUMPING INSULIN

PREVENTING AND SOLVING PUMP PROBLEMS

15

In this chapter, we:

- identify problems that can occur when using a pump,
- troubleshoot unexpected high blood sugars caused by a pump,
- show how to lower risks for pump problems, and
- review when to call your physician/health care team.

An insulin pump enhances your ability to maintain good control, but it is also a mechanical device that can cause control problems. Maintenance and monitoring are needed to ensure that a pump is working. Most pump problems occur in the first six months of use, then decrease in frequency as you become experienced. As you learn how to troubleshoot situations like unexpected high blood sugars, these problems tend to decrease in frequency and severity.

Keep in mind that the first sign of a pump problem is often an **unexpected high blood sugar**. If you have a high blood sugar, don't blindly assume you have misjudged or miscalculated your insulin requirements. Remember to use an injection of Regular insulin if you have **any suspicion** that your pump is not delivering insulin. Start using injections whenever two consecutive unexpected high blood sugars occur. Stay on injections until the source of the problem is found.

TROUBLESHOOTING THE PUMP

An insulin pump is a mechanical device that can fail due to improper technique or defective parts. The pump sets off an audible alarm for only some of these problems as outlined in Table 15.1 on the next page. **Keep your ear open for pump alarms and keep your eye open for unexplained high blood sugars.** A high blood sugar is seen within 2 to 4 hours if insulin delivery is interrupted for any reason. If your blood sugars are unexpectedly high or are over 250 mg/dl on two consecutive tests, **take an injection to reduce the high blood sugar before troubleshooting the pump**.

Test for ketones in the urine. If ketones are present at moderate or large levels, contact your physician/health care team. They may recommend giving 50 to 100 % more insulin than normal **by injection** to lower the blood sugar level. Check blood sugars hourly until corrected. If you are unsure of the reason for high blood sugars, take Regular insulin by injection and replace the reservoir and infusion set, using a new injection site, as precautions. Table 15.1 outlines some common pump problems and what to do about them.

Table 15.1 How To Detect And Fix Pump Problems

Problem	What To Do For It	Will Pump Alarm?
leak between the O-rings	Look for bubbles, mist or fluid between the O-rings in the reservoir. If any of these is seen, replace the reservoir. Though the amount of insulin between the O-rings seems small, the effect on blood sugars can be great.	No
unprimed infusion line	Prime the infusion line.	No
empty reservoir	Replace with a newly filled reservoir.	Yes
dislodged needle/Sof-Set	Reinsert needle with sterile technique, or replace Sof-Set.	No
clog	Difficult to see, a clog may appear as a white, crystalline deposit in the tubing. As it develops, insulin is lost on the infusion tubing and may create high blood sugars. If a clog is present, replace the entire infusion set.	Yes
hematoma at the infusion site	If a lump can be felt beneath the skin at the infusion site or discomfort is present, subcutaneous bleeding is likely. Place the infusion site in a new location.	No
blood in the infusion tubing	Replace the infusion set at a new location.	No
incorrect programming	Check the programming. If you have improperly programmed the pump, reprogram it.	No
weak or dead battery	If a low battery warning occurs, replace the battery.	Yes
mechanical problem	Insulin pumps have several safety alarms. If an alarm occurs, refer to your pump manual. Then contact your pump company, if necessary, to remedy the problem.	Yes

REDUCING RISKS FOR PUMP PROBLEMS

Ways to reduce the risk of running out of insulin, clogging and leaking are covered below:

RUNNING DRY

Most reservoirs today can hold 300 units of insulin when filled. Many pumpers forget how quickly this insulin disappears. The following tips help in managing your insulin supply:

- To keep from running out of insulin at an inconvenient time, **plan ahead**. Have a regular schedule for changing your infusion site and filling your reservoir. Choose a time that is convenient for you, and change your site every second day at that same time. Change infusion sets in the morning to avoid having a dislodged needle or other mechanical problem go undetected for several hours while asleep.
- If you've used more insulin than usual and don't have enough in your reservoir to last until your next scheduled change, conserve the insulin in your pump by using

injections from a syringe for all boluses. Use the remaining insulin in your pump to continue your basal rate, making sure there is enough insulin left in your reservoir to do this. Keep syringes available for situations like this.

- If you run out of insulin in your reservoir and have **no other insulin available**, remember that a pump with an empty reservoir has **17 to 25 units left in the infusion line**. After clamping your infusion line, use sterile technique to disconnect your infusion line from your syringe. Fill your syringe with air by pulling the plunger back, replace this air-filled syringe into your pump, prime the pump so that you make contact between the drive mechanism and plunger (so air will come out of the syringe), and then reconnect the syringe very snugly to your infusion line.

  Now program your pump normally. Although you no longer have insulin in your reservoir, the insulin in your infusion line will be pushed by air through the infusion line and made available for use. **Extra** blood sugar checks will need to be done because this method of delivering insulin is **not reliable**. Use this method **only for emergencies until new supplies are available.** Discuss this method with your physician/health care team before trying it.

CLOGGING

A frequent cause of clogged lines comes from using the wrong type of Regular insulin. Insulin is a crystalline substance held in solution by buffering. If the buffer is inappropriate for use in a plastic infusion line, the insulin will precipitate inside the line and begin to close it off. Clogging then occurs and you are no longer getting insulin.

The best way to prevent clogging is to use an insulin with a phosphate buffer. The insulin with the fewest clogging problems is Velosulin®, a human Regular insulin made by Nordisk™. If clogging problems occur and you are using another insulin, discuss changing brands with your physician/health care team. Some pumpers notice less clogging when using infusion sets with tubing that is more insulin-compatible, such as polyolefin (Polyfin®). If you are using another type of tubing, consider changing to Polyfin®. If you are experiencing frequent clogging, such as more than once a month, check that you are using a compatible insulin in your pump and proper infusion sets. When clogging occurs, you are losing insulin on the inside of your infusion set. After changing to Velosulin or to a polyolefin infusion set, you will begin to receive all the insulin your pump sends and may need **less insulin**.

There are other possible causes for clogged lines. Poor technique when changing the reservoir and infusion set can cause clogging. Foreign materials such as betadine or alcohol may cause clogging, if introduced into the reservoir or line. Although unlikely, certain items, such as hand lotions, hair sprays, paints and solvents, which are on your hands, skin, clothing or in the air, may penetrate the infusion tubing and cause clogging. Always use special care when handling your insulin, syringes and infusion sets. If the tubing comes in contact with very hot water, as in a steaming shower or hot tub, the heat may coagulate the insulin. **Protect your insulin from heat.**

If you try to give a large bolus through a clogged line, an alarm should sound on the pump. But if you give only a small bolus or have only basal insulin passing through the line, an alarm will not sound until pressure has built up. Depending on the situation, this delay in warning could be several hours. Before you get an alarm to warn you, your blood sugar may already be high.

A common sign of clogging is a high blood sugar.

LEAKING

Insulin leaking from your reservoir or infusion set is difficult to see or feel. The amount of insulin lost is so small it is quite hard to detect and your pump will not warn you of leaks. **Regular blood sugar tests are usually the only way to detect leaks.** As with clogs:

The most common sign of a leak is a high blood sugar.

HOW TO CHECK FOR LEAKS AND CLOGS

If an unexpected high blood sugar occurs, **remove the infusion set** and:

- Send a 2 unit bolus through the tubing to check for **clogs**. If no insulin appears at the tip, the infusion set is clogged. If insulin appears **immediately** at the tip, the infusion set is not clogged.
- If you are using an infusion set with a needle, insert the needle into a bar of soap to intentionally clog it. Send another 2 unit bolus through, then check the infusion line, hub and O-rings for **leaks**. If insulin can be seen or smelled at the hub or is visible along the infusion line or between the O-rings, a leak is responsible for the high blood sugars.
- If neither a clog nor leak is present, consider other causes for high blood sugars.

Whenever your blood sugar is high, sort out in your mind whether there is a clear cause for it, such as extra carbohydrate intake, too little bolus or basal insulin, an infection, etc.. If there is not a clear reason for the high reading, use Table 15.2 to check for leaks. The quickest way to tell whether a clog or leak has caused a high blood sugar is to remove the needle from your skin and test your equipment.

**Remember: frequent blood sugar testing
warns you of problems before they become serious!**

Table 15.2 How To Detect And Prevent Leaks	
Source of Leak	**Remedy**
between the O-rings in the reservoir	Look between the O-rings. If you see any fluid, bubbles or mist between the O-rings, replace the reservoir immediately.
at the hub that connects the reservoir and infusion set	Look for liquid in the hub. Then smell the hub. Velosulin has a distinctive odor like creosote. If an odor is present, a leak is likely. If you have trouble tightening the infusion set to the luer lock, try tweezers or any device that grips but does not damage.
hole or tear in the infusion line	Inspect the infusion line after giving a bolus. If a bead of insulin appears on the infusion line or where the line attaches to the needle, a leak has occured. Protect your infusion line by careful maneuvering around children, pets, zippers and sharp objects.
dislodged needle or Sof-Set cannula	Carefully check the infusion site for a dislodged needle or cannula. This may be caused by strenuous movements, sweating, or ineffective tape or adhesive. Use Micropore® tape or Tegaderm HP® to secure bent metal needles. Always secure a safety loop with extra tape.

Do not continue to use your pump if your blood sugars remain high. If you are unable to correct an elevated blood sugar while using your pump, **stop using it**. Anytime your blood sugar readings are over 250 mg/dl twice in a row without a good reason, replace your syringe and infusion set immediately, take a conventional injection of Regular insulin and test your blood sugar more often to make sure you have corrected the problem. Check your urine for ketones; call your physician/health care team immediately if ketones are moderate or high.

UNEXPLAINED HIGH BLOOD SUGARS:

- Give insulin by syringe until the cause is identified and corrected.
- Sliding scale doses can be determined from the information in Table 7.1. If a rapid lowering of the blood sugar is desired, a quicker fall is usually seen with an intramuscular (IM) injection of Regular insulin.[79] Discuss this with your physician. Intramuscular injections can be given with a standard insulin syringe into the inner thigh or biceps, although those with more subcutaneous fat have to select an IM injection site carefully.
- If moderate or large ketones are present in the urine, insulin doses that normally would be used to lower a high blood sugar may need to be increased by as much as 50% to 100%. Again, discuss this with your physician. Check your blood sugar readings every hour until blood sugar control is regained.
- Drink large amounts of water or other noncaloric fluid with an intake of at least 8 oz. every 30 minutes until the blood sugar is normal. This helps the kidneys rid the body of excess sugar. Sports drinks, like Gatorade, or water with a pinch of potassium-based No Salt®, can be used to replace potassium in early ketoacidosis.
- If nausea occurs, call your physician immediately. If vomiting occurs, call your physician immediately and go to an emergency room. When nausea is caused by ketoacidosis, it is very serious and can cause death.

If a severe insulin reaction or ketoacidosis occurs, this should always raise a red flag. The absence of a clear reason, such as an infection, indicates that insulin doses are incorrect, the pump has run dry, is leaking or clogging, or that the basic principles of blood sugar control are not understood. Discuss this problem with your physician/health care team to resolve it and prevent it from happening again.

"Little minds are interested in the extraordinary; great minds in the commonplace."

Elbert Hubbard

PREVENTING AND SOLVING
SKIN PROBLEMS

16

An infusion needle is like a splinter or any other foreign body placed under the skin. It can cause irritation, discomfort or infection. Skin problems can also be caused by the adhesive material used to tape the needle or infusion set to the skin, or more rarely by insulin itself. Some pumpers have no difficulty with skin problems, while others have to pay close attention to avoid them.

Who is likely to develop skin problems? No one really knows. No clear relationship exists between how well blood sugars are controlled and skin problems associated with pump use. The wise choice is to follow safe techniques to reduce your risk.

This chapter discusses how to deal with infusion site problems:

- tape allergies,
- infections,
- bleeding,
- pump bumps, and
- pump hypertrophy.

TAPE ALLERGIES

Your skin may not accept every tape or dressing you use to keep the infusion set in place. A particular tape may cause an allergic reaction. This problem is easy to diagnose because the redness that is seen on the skin patterns itself after the shape of the tape or dressing. Itching or irritation will accompany this allergic reaction.

If you are allergic to a tape, the allergy will usually occur a few days or weeks after the tape is first used. To treat a tape allergy, switch to another brand of tape or adhesive dressing. The tape that sticks best is Micropore® skin tape by 3M. If a problem occurs with white Micropore® tape, brown Micropore® tape is less likely to cause allergies. Silk tape can also be used. Other tapes are less effective at staying in place while swimming or showering, or leave adhesive behind on the skin.

Another treatment for a tape allergy is to use protective dressing, such as Skin Prep®, on the skin before applying the tape. This product provides a protective barrier between the skin and the offending tape and can often reduce or prevent the risk of an allergic reaction. Discuss using Skin Prep® or changing to another tape with your physician/health care team.

INFECTIONS

The risk for infection increases in using an insulin pump. Most infections result from poor technique, such as breathing onto the infusion set, touching the infusion needle or top of the insulin bottle, not using Betadine® Solution or Hibiclens® on the skin, or leaving the infusion set at one site longer than 48 hours. A good way to prevent infections is to assume they will happen and then take care that they don't.

Watch for these signs of an infection at the infusion site:

- redness or inflammation,
- warmth,
- pain, and
- swelling.

If any of these signs occur at the infusion site, contact your physician/health care team immediately. An early infection is easy to treat with an antibiotic. If treatment is delayed, an infection **can develop into an abscess and require surgery or hospitalization**.

When you have an infection, that infection can spread to any new infusion site. If you have an infection or suspect one, remove the infusion set you are using and start injecting your insulin **with a syringe**. Use a new infusion set at a new site only after you have started an antibiotic. **Never** reuse an infusion set removed from an infected site.

Your physician will be far happier calling in a prescription for you than having to lance an abscess or write hospital admission orders. You will also be assuring your physician that you are a well-informed, well-trained pump user when you call your physician at the first sign of this potentially serious problem. Do not wait until it has become a crisis.

PREVENTING INFECTIONS

The most important factor in preventing infections is good technique in preparing your pump and infusion site. Bacteria are usually transferred by touch or through the breath. They grow naturally on the skin, but sterile technique can reduce the number of bacteria on the skin at the infusion site, and you can prevent transferring bacteria to this area or the infusion set through touch. Sterile technique means not allowing your syringe, infusion set or needle to touch anything. Sterile technique means eliminating bacteria already present on your skin at the infusion site, and preventing contact between your washed hands or sterile equipment and any bacteria. Review the techniques outlined on pages 22 through 24 to avoid infections at the infusion site.

BLEEDING

Bleeding from a broken blood vessel can occur whenever a needle is placed into the skin. Because the needle in an infusion set stays in the skin for 48 hours and may move slightly when you dance, ride a bike or bump into the kitchen counter, bleeding occurs more often with a pump than with injections. Fortunately, bleeding is infrequent and usually creates a cosmetic problem, not a health problem. Bleeding can occur in three areas:

1. Onto the Skin

This is noticed as blood stains on the skin beneath the tape or dressing. The infusion needle causes this problem when it nicks a tiny blood vessel near the surface of the skin. Some pumpers ignore this situation as long as the site is not inflamed, painful, enlarged, or threatening to discolor their wardrobe. Monitor this situation carefully to make sure it doesn't worsen. Even though this situation isn't critical, moving the infusion site ensures that further bleeding will not occur.

2. Inside the Needle

This is noticed as blood inside the infusion tubing near the needle. In this situation, there may be enough bleeding at the tip of the needle under the skin to dilute the insulin the pump is delivering. Diluting the insulin within a pool of blood often destroys its action. A high blood sugar may be the first sign of this problem. Any movement of the needle due to motion or rubbing may increase bleeding and make the insulin less likely to work.

**Whenever you see any blood inside the infusion tubing,
immediately sterilize the needle (pg. 23) and move it to a new site.**

3. Under the Skin

Bleeding under the skin may cause a hematoma which is usually noticed as a lump under the skin at the infusion site. As you touch the infusion site, it feels like a hard lump about the size of a quarter underneath the needle. A hematoma can feel uncomfortable or sore in the same way that a bruise can. The skin may be normal in color or slightly red. Bleeding into the infusion tubing or around the needle on your skin may accompany a hematoma.

This pool of blood dilutes the insulin the pump is delivering. Again, a high blood sugar may be the first sign of this problem. A pool of blood is also an invitation to bacteria to grow and multiply, increasing the risk for infection. The infusion needle is a foreign body; if bacteria are present on the needle, they can multiply within the hematoma and cause an abscess. Monitor the site carefully. If you have any doubts or questions about whether a sore spot is a hematoma or an infection, call your physician/health care team immediately. Early treatment is always best.

Move the infusion site immediately if you find a hard, enlarged spot under the skin.

Pump Bumps

A pump bump sounds like a dent found in your pump after you've dropped it. Instead, it is a slightly reddish, raised, pimple-sized spot found at the needle site after the needle has been in place for 48 hours. It often itches. After changing the infusion set and moving the needle to a new site, the bump gradually disappears. Several theories have been proposed as causes for pump bumps, including a reaction to the coatings on the outside of the needle or a reaction to preservatives and other trace chemicals found in the insulin itself.

If you are concerned about pump bumps for cosmetic reasons, there are a couple of ways to reduce the chances of getting them. Methods recommended already are to cover the infusion site with Betadine® before inserting the infusion needle, to take extra care to use sterile technique, and to change the infusion site regularly every 48 hours.

Any improvements in healing or the responsiveness of the immune system also help. Normal blood sugars are critical for quick healing, but this can be aided somewhat by vitamin supplements, including an antioxidant complex and 25 mg. of chelated zinc a day.

Another way to reduce chances for pump bumps is to be sure the needle has been taped securely to the skin, so that less shifting of the needle occurs during movement and bending.

Another method is to switch from needles to Sof-Sets® which are made of teflon and do not react with the skin. This may decrease pump bumps and other types of irritation. Teflon catheters do not have the same coating as needle catheters. Reports from pumpers who were bothered by pump bumps suggest some reduction after switching to Sof-Sets®.

If using a Sof-Set®, it is important to secure it firmly to the skin to prevent kinking of the teflon catheter. For better sticking and to decrease the likelihood of an infection, we recommend first applying betadine to the skin, letting it dry, and then placing a 3" piece of Micropore® tape over the betadine at the intended infusion site. The white cover tab is removed from the Sof-Set®, but be sure to leave the tan tab in place. To avoid crimping of the teflon cannula, use a fast hand motion to **quickly** insert the Sof-Set® through the Micropore® tape. Then secure it to the tape underneath with the transparent dressing provided with the Sof-Set®.

If you have an allergy to Micropore™ tape, either Caraskin® or Polyskin® can also be used. Because only the soft teflon is left under the skin, there is nothing to warn you if it comes out of the skin or has kinked. The greater ease with which Sof-Sets® become kinked or displaced requires **frequent blood sugar monitoring**. If irregular blood sugar results are seen when using Sof-Sets®, it may be better to use metal needles and deal with the pump bumps in another way.

These simple techniques can help reduce pump bump problems. If pump bumps do occur, a small amount of Neosporin®, Bacitracin® or other antibiotic salve found at any local pharmacy will decrease the irritation and speed their disappearance.

HYPERTROPHY AT THE INFUSION SITE

Some pumpers find that after using their pump for some time, a slight enlargement occurs in the area of the body where the infusion needle is placed. Since hypertrophy is a medical term that describes an enlargement (atrophy is its opposite), this is called pump hypertrophy.

Pump hypertrophy may be caused by the higher concentrations of insulin placed under the skin at the infusion site. This extra insulin causes growth to occur among the cells in contact with the insulin. This causes no medical problems, although some find it a cosmetic concern. Don't be alarmed if you notice this in the area of your infusion sites. Discuss this with your physician/health care team if you feel it is a problem. If pump hypertrophy or pump bumps occur, you should avoid these areas for 3 or 4 weeks. Temporarily switch to other areas of the body, such as the buttocks, to allow healing to occur.

"Never go to bed mad. Stay up and fight."

Phyllis Diller

PUMPING INSULIN

BLOOD SUGAR PATTERNS AND WHAT TO DO ABOUT THEM

17

Recognizing the patterns in your blood sugars is essential to control, but many pumpers have difficulty identifying these patterns. Some typical patterns are shown in the Diabetes Advanced Workshop charts below. These patterns can occur on several days' charts each week (repeated), or once in a while (occasional). Possible solutions to these problem patterns are suggested. If the chart pattern is repeated and the suggested solution(s) works, the suggested solution(s) should be incorporated into your blood sugar management on an ongoing basis. If the pattern is occasional, the solution is a one-time fix that can be reused in the future if the pattern occurs again.

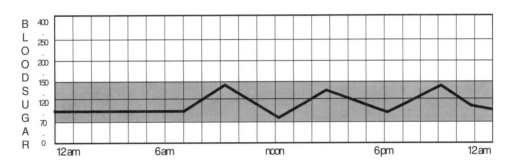

PATTERN: NORMAL
WHAT TO DO: Keep up the great work!

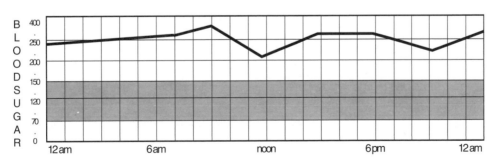

PATTERN: HIGH
WHAT TO DO: Raise basal rates and boluses. Review diet, exercise & weight for improvements. ?infection ?pain ?stress ?bad insulin, etc.

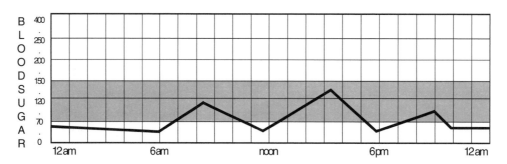

PATTERN: Low

WHAT TO DO: Lower basal rates and/or boluses, eat more carbohydrate.

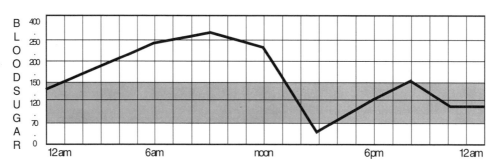

PATTERN: HIGH-LOW

WHAT TO DO: Lower High Blood Sugar Bolus, eat before blood sugar drops.

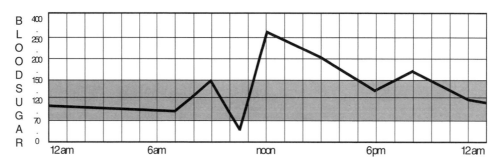

PATTERN: LOW-HIGH

WHAT TO DO: Use glucose or Sweet Tarts®, eat less for lows.

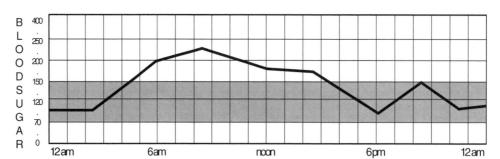

PATTERN: DAWN PHENOMENON

WHAT TO DO: Increase early morning basal rate, usually at 1 to 3 a.m.

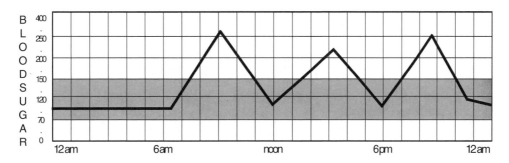

PATTERN: SPIKES BETWEEN MEALS

WHAT TO DO: Take meal bolus earlier, split meal, eat lower glycemic index foods, add fiber (psyllium and/or guar gum) before the meal.

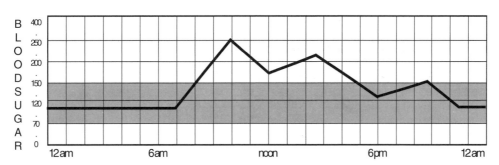

PATTERN: HIGH AFTER A MEAL

WHAT TO DO: Raise meal bolus, less carbohydrate, exercise after meal.

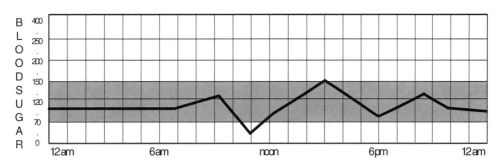

PATTERN: LOW AFTER A MEAL

WHAT TO DO: Lower meal bolus, increase carbohydrate.

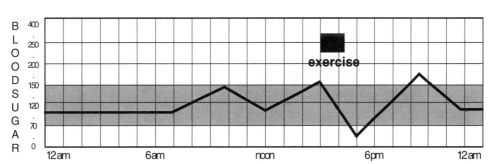

PATTERN: EXERCISE LOWS

WHAT TO DO: Lower insulin, increase carbohydrate.

SOLVING HIGH BLOOD SUGARS BEFORE AND AFTER BREAKFAST

18

The first blood sugar of the day can be the hardest to control, especially if you have a Dawn Phenomenon. Waking up with a high blood sugar after going to bed with a normal reading is very discouraging. A blood sugar that creeps up after breakfast for no clear reason is also annoying.

This chapter presents:

- causes and corrections for high blood sugars before breakfast, and
- causes and corrections for high blood sugars after breakfast.

WHAT TO DO FOR HIGH BLOOD SUGARS BEFORE BREAKFAST

When the waking blood sugar is high, control for the rest of the day becomes hard. Why does a high morning blood sugar throw off the rest of the day? Because the insulin level in the blood is low. This allows the liver to start producing more sugar! Once the liver begins this process of making sugar and releasing it into the bloodstream, the liver becomes difficult to stop and creates a magnified rise in the blood sugar after breakfast. Extra insulin is required to stop the liver and bring the blood sugar back down.

Complicating this situation, when extra insulin has been taken at breakfast and lunch to lower the blood sugar, insulin reactions in the late afternoon and early evening become likely. Excess food eaten in the panic of the reaction can then cause the blood sugar to rise again with a repetition of the cycle. **When blood sugars are high in the morning, be careful of afternoon lows. When several High Blood Sugar Boluses are taken to lower high blood sugars in the morning, an insulin reaction later in the day becomes likely.**

On the next few pages are five common causes for high blood sugars before breakfast, followed by four causes for highs after breakfast. Tips for actions to take to correct these problems are also provided.

1. TOO LITTLE BASAL INSULIN

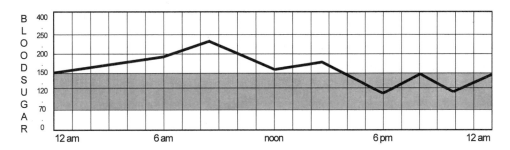

This chart shows a blood sugar rising during the night because the basal rate is set **too low**. When too little basal insulin is delivered, the sugar rises in the blood because it is unable to enter cells where it's needed.

Tests and Results:

To discover if your high morning blood sugar is caused by too little basal insulin, test the blood sugar at these times and look for these results:

Bedtime: Normal blood sugar.
3 a.m.: Usually midway between the bedtime and waking blood sugars.
Waking: Always higher than the 3 a.m. and bedtime readings.

Pattern Frequency:

Happens regularly when the overnight basal rate is set too low.

What To Do:

Raise the basal rate slightly during the night as described in Chapter 8 and test this rate as described in Table 8.1. Be careful when raising the basal rate. Test blood sugars more often. When insulin levels are low, excess glucose is being produced by the liver. This may require a lot of insulin early in the day, but if too much insulin is used, a reaction later in the day results.

2. HIGH PROTEIN DINNER

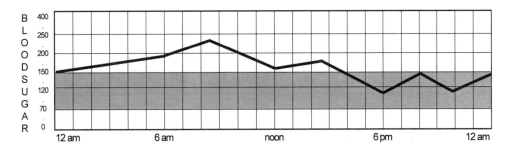

This pattern is identical to the previous one, but the cause and treatment are quite different. When protein is eaten, 40% to 50% of it will change slowly into glucose over a period of several hours following the meal. The protein in most meals has little influence on blood sugar levels, but when lots of protein is eaten it can cause an overnight rise in blood sugars. Some examples of heavy protein intake are an 8 to 12 ounce steak, a Mexican dinner with a lot of refried beans, or an evening snack of a half pound of peanuts.

Tests and Results:

To discover if your high morning blood sugar is caused by a high protein dinner, test at these times and look for these results:

Bedtime:	Normal blood sugar
3 a.m.:	Usually midway between the bedtime and waking blood sugars.
Waking:	Always higher than the 3 a.m. and bedtime readings.

Pattern Frequency:

Uncommon, occurs only after a meal containing an excess of protein.

What To Do:

1. An obvious solution is to limit the protein in the evening meal.
2. Another alternative is raising the basal rate slightly overnight to offset the increased production of glucose from the extra protein. If your pump has a temporary basal rate, use this feature. If your pump does not have this feature, change the basal rate, but **be sure to return it back to its normal setting in the morning**.
3. Also possible is waking up halfway through the night, checking the blood sugar and correcting with a high blood sugar bolus, if needed, at that time.

The second method can be used if the same high protein meal is eaten regularly and a pumper knows this meal always raises the blood sugar overnight. The third method is best to use when experience is limited and a nighttime insulin reaction is to be avoided.

3. HIGH BEDTIME BLOOD SUGAR

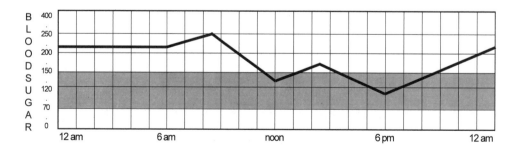

This pattern is easy to identify. As can be seen, the morning blood sugar ends up being high because the blood sugar was already high the night before at bedtime.

Tests and Results:

To determine if a high morning blood sugar is caused by going to bed with a high blood sugar, blood sugar tests are done at these times, with these anticipated results:

Bedtime: High
3 a.m.:   High
Waking: High

Pattern Frequency:

Varies from person to person; occurs more often if the bedtime blood sugar is not tested regularly. It is also frequent if the evening meal and evening snacks are not covered with enough Carbohydrate Bolus, or a high bedtime blood sugar is not covered with enough High Blood Sugar Bolus, due to fear of a nighttime reaction.

What To Do:

After the night basal has been tested and correctly set, fully cover the carbohydrate eaten during the evening hours. When the blood sugar is high at bedtime, take a bolus large enough to bring it down, but small enough to avoid a nighttime reaction. Be cautious and test regularly, especially at bedtime. A test at 1 a.m. or 2 a.m. helps in avoiding nighttime low blood sugars. If you are having frequent or severe reactions during the night, or are concerned about having night reactions, be sure to discuss this with your physician/health care team.

4. DAWN PHENOMENON

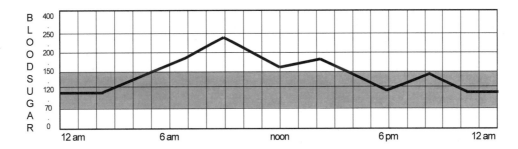

Discussed in Chapter 7, the Dawn Phenomenon pattern shows the need for an increased basal rate, starting between the hours of 1 a.m. and 3 a.m. for those who sleep standard hours.

Tests and Results:

To discover if your high morning blood sugar is caused by a Dawn Phenomenon, test at these times and look for these results:

Bedtime: Normal blood sugar.
2 a.m.:   Close to the bedtime blood sugar, lower than the waking reading.
Waking: Higher than the 2 a.m. and bedtime readings.

Pattern Frequency:

Of those using pumps, 50% to 70% will need an increased basal rate beginning between 1 a.m. and 3 a.m. Be sure to check with your physician/health care team to make sure you have a Dawn Phenomenon **before** increasing your basal rate in the early morning hours.

What To Do:

Raise the basal rate starting at 1 a.m. to 3 a.m., or one to two hours before the time the blood sugar usually begins to rise. A lead time of 90 to 120 minutes is needed for the increased basal rate to begin raising the insulin level in the blood stream.

A good rule of thumb is that a smaller increase in the basal rate will be needed when the increase in basal rate is started earlier. If you find that your basal has to be raised by 0.5 u/hr (say from 0.5 to 1.0 u/hr) at 4 a.m. to prevent a high waking blood sugar, you can often get a better result by increasing the basal rate from 0.5 u/hr to only 0.6 or 0.7 u/hr at 1 a.m. or 2 a.m.

5. OVERTREATING A NIGHTTIME INSULIN REACTION

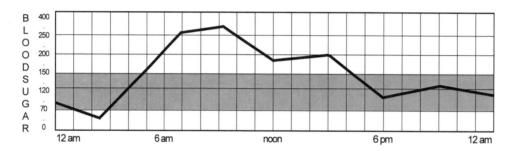

It's hard to be rational after waking from the release of stress hormones in the middle of the night. During a low blood sugar, brain cells aren't getting enough fuel to operate well. In the fear and confusion that follows, emptying the refrigerator seems perfectly normal and reassuring.

This overeating, however, results in sky-high blood sugars in the morning, especially following the release of excessive levels of stress hormones into the bloodstream. Blood sugars may continue to stay high for several hours into the day, as a result of the stress hormone release.

Tests and Results:

To discover if your high morning blood sugar is caused by overtreating a nighttime insulin reaction, test at these times and look for these results:

Bedtime:	Varies: can be low, normal or high.
Night:	Low to very low.
Waking:	Always high after eating too much.

Pattern Frequency:

Happens whenever too much is eaten for a nighttime reaction. Nighttime reactions are common when the night basal is set too high, after heavy exercise, when the bolus for dinner is too large, or if a bedtime high blood sugar has been covered with too much insulin.

112

What To Do:

The best solution is to determine why the nighttime reactions are occurring and avoid them. The second best solution is to keep glucose tablets or Sweet Tarts® beside the bed and use them routinely to treat reactions. Even in the midst of a nighttime reaction, it is hard to overdose on glucose tablets.

A NOTE ABOUT SOMOYGI REACTIONS:

The Somoygi reaction is named after Michael Somoygi, who first proposed this theory in 1959. His theory was that a high waking blood sugar could result from sleeping through an insulin reaction during the night.

According to his theory, nighttime low blood sugars, by triggering stress hormone release, would cause high blood sugars on waking even though nothing was eaten for the reaction. Research has shown, however, that if the Somoygi reaction does occur it rarely causes the waking blood sugar to be high.

Most researchers favor the view that high morning blood sugars are not caused by night reactions. After sleeping through a reaction, the blood sugar the next morning is usually 50 to 150 mg/dl. Because of the higher stress hormone levels, blood sugars, however, often rise after breakfast.

Generally the morning blood sugar will be no higher than 150 after sleeping through a nighttime reaction, **unless** the early morning basal rate is too low. Here, the release of stress hormones combined with too little basal insulin can cause a high waking sugar. If you have high blood sugars in the morning and blame them on reactions during sleep, test your blood sugar at 2 a.m. to rule out a reaction and carefully consider other causes.

Unrecognized nighttime reactions, though they rarely cause high waking blood sugars, can occur frequently. See Chapter 13 for the signs that suggest this is happening. To stop nighttime reactions, carefully consider whether excess insulin is coming from a high dinner bolus or from a night basal that is set too high. Decrease the insulin that is excessive. Start by retesting the night basal rate as shown in Table 8.1.

You may find that you are having both the Dawn Phenomenon and occasional nighttime reactions. If this is happening, you will want to decrease the basal in the first part of the night to prevent the insulin reactions. You may need to increase it in the early morning to prevent a blood sugar rise from the Dawn Phenomenon.

Keep in mind that if you are having any of the mechanical problems outlined in Chapter 15, these can also occur during the night and cause your morning blood sugar to be elevated. Mechanical problems, however, tend to be random and with good technique will never cause consistently high morning blood sugars.

What To Do For High Blood Sugars After Breakfast

It is also possible to wake up with a normal blood sugar in the morning, but then lose control when it rises sharply after breakfast. Four common causes for this are discussed below.

1. Too Little Breakfast Bolus

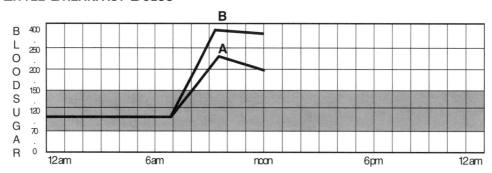

Here the breakfast bolus is too little for the carbohydrate eaten (line A), or the bolus for breakfast was forgotten altogether (line B).

Pattern Frequency:

Very frequent if the ratio of insulin to carbohydrate is too low (i.e., not enough insulin for the food eaten). It is infrequent if the amount of carbohydrate is misjudged in unusual circumstances, such as when eating out, and infrequent (we hope) if the bolus was forgotten.

What To Do:

Recheck the ratio of a unit of insulin to grams of carbohydrate (see Chapter 10) if this is happening frequently. Review how to measure the carbohydrate in any meal that seems to consistently give you a problem.

2. Unrecognized Nighttime Reaction

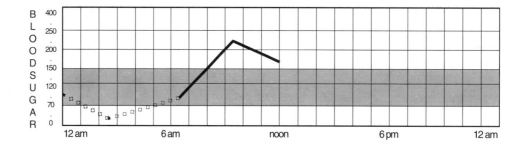

The pattern above is typical for the morning after an unrecognized nighttime reaction. Some low blood sugars may occur without significant stress hormone release, but for this particular blood sugar response, significant amounts of stress hormones **must** be released. Review Chapter 13 for signs of nighttime reactions.

When the basal rate is correctly set, a release of stress hormones from a nighttime reaction is unlikely to raise the waking blood sugar. But after eating a normal amount of carbohydrate for breakfast, the usually adequate bolus of insulin is blunted and the blood sugar rises. Because stress hormones can raise blood sugar levels for 8 to 10 hours after a major reaction, the blood sugar may stay high at lunch and into the afternoon as well.

Pattern Frequency:

It varies from individual to individual. Most people who have nighttime insulin reactions appear to sleep through most of them. Remember: the only reactions you remember are those that wake you up.

What To Do:

Recognize that insulin reactions may be occurring and correct the cause or causes if they are. Review Chapter 13 for signs of nighttime reactions. Set your clock to wake you up at 2 a.m. and check your blood sugar.

3. BREAKFAST BOLUS TAKEN TOO CLOSE TO THE MEAL

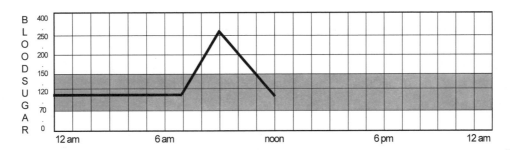

Boluses of insulin take at least 15 minutes to have any effect, and 2 to 3 hours before they begin to peak in their action. After eating carbohydrate, the blood sugar begins to immediately rise. When a bolus is taken just before a meal, the carbohydrate will raise the blood sugar before the late bolus has a chance to counteract it. A high blood sugar follows. This high blood sugar then returns to normal before lunch, as the insulin finally has its desired effect.

Pattern Frequency:

It depends on the individual's response to insulin, the amount of carbohydrate eaten, activity levels after the meal, and glycemic indexes of the foods eaten.

What To Do:

Take the bolus 30 to 45 minutes before eating, eat less carbohydrate for breakfast and add a mid-morning carbohydrate snack, take some fiber like psyllium or guar gum before having breakfast, or get extra exercise just after breakfast.

4. HIGH GLYCEMIC INDEX FOOD EATEN AT BREAKFAST

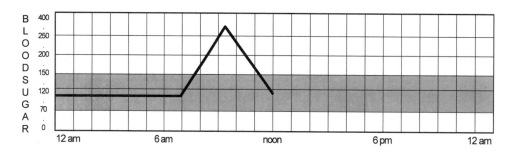

This pattern is identical to that for a breakfast bolus taken too close to the meal. But instead of taking the breakfast bolus too late, a fast-acting carbohydrate has spiked the blood sugar while the insulin was more slowly entering the blood. As discussed in Chapter 6, some foods have a high glycemic index and will cause a greater rise in the blood sugar after meals, even though no more carbohydrate than usual was eaten.

If someone has 50 grams of carbohydrate for breakfast, but eats this as ripe bananas, yogurt with fruit syrup mixed in the bottom of the container, or toasted cheese sandwiches, a spike in the post-breakfast blood sugar is typical.

Frequency:

It depends on the glycemic index of the foods eaten and on the response of the person eating these particular foods.

What To Do:

Check the glycemic index of the suspected food in Appendix B. Partially or totally replace the suspect food with another food known to have a low glycemic index (old-fashioned oatmeal, Cheerios™, strawberries, plain yogurt with fresh fruit sliced into it). Other solutions include taking the bolus earlier before eating, eating less carbohydrate for breakfast while adding a mid-morning carbohydrate snack, taking some fiber like psyllium or guar gum before eating breakfast, or getting extra exercise just after breakfast.

The graphs above illustrate most of the reasons for high blood sugars during the morning hours. Some of these problems, such as too little Carbohydrate Bolus, a high protein meal, a bolus taken too close to the meal, and high glycemic index foods, can occur at other meals of the day. The solutions above will work for the same problems occurring at other meals.

"The advantage of emotions is that they lead us astray."

Oscar Wilde

Pumping Insulin

Controlling Variable Blood Sugars

19

Variable blood sugars can happen even when using an insulin pump. Though a pump provides the best opportunity for stable, normal blood sugars, it does not guarantee this. "Variable" is hard to define. Blood sugar readings that one pumper considers poor control might be a significant improvement for another. Most people would would be annoyed by blood sugars that frequently stray outside the 70 to 140 mg/dl range before meals and beyond 200 mg/dl after meals. If they **show very little pattern when they do this**, they are variable.

If blood sugars are often high at a certain time of day, such as bedtime, this is not a variable pattern, but a consistently abnormal pattern. With a consistently abnormal pattern, the cause is usually easy to identify. It may be that the Carbohydrate Bolus is too small for the evening meal, or there's a problem with snacking after dinner, or the basal rate is set too low.

Truly variable blood sugars, on the other hand, have little identifiable pattern to them. They do, however, have causes that turn out to be variable and random, such as stress or exercise that occurs intermittently. These causes for variable blood sugars can usually be identified.

This chapter deals with some factors that cause variable blood sugars, including:

- insulin reactions,
- a variable lifestyle,
- problems with carbohydrates, and
- stress.

Questions To Ask When There Is Poor Control But No Pattern:

If there is **no apparent pattern** in your blood sugars and your control is not what you would like, check for the following:

• Frequent or severe low blood sugars?	yes	no
• Erratic eating (different carbs, different times)?	yes	no
• Skipped meals?	yes	no
• Insulin doses that change a lot from day to day?	yes	no
• Exercise that varies in timing, duration & intensity?	yes	no
• No exercise at all?	yes	no
• Irregular sleep hours?	yes	no
• Stress?	yes	no

If you answer "yes" several times, your control can be improved by dealing with these areas of your life. As you introduce more regularity into your life and prevent lows and lessen stress, your charts will begin to have a recognizable pattern to them. If this pattern does not show the control you would like, at least you can then analyze it for solutions.

INSULIN REACTIONS

For some people, **frequent insulin reactions are often a cause for blood sugar variability**. If too much insulin is being taken or if the reaction is overtreated in a panic, variable blood sugars result. If a high blood sugar occurs because the reaction was overtreated and extra bolus insulin is needed, this increases the risk for another reaction.

PATTERN:

Insulin reactions as a cause of variable blood sugars are easy to recognize on charts: a pattern of frequent low blood sugars that are followed 1 to 4 hours later by unusual highs. When low blood sugars are shortly followed by blood sugars above 150 mg/dl, overtreatment is likely. If the highs are then followed in the next few hours by another low, too much insulin is being given, usually in the High Blood Sugar Bolus used to bring the blood sugar down.

WHAT TO DO:

- Use glucose tablets or Sweet Tarts® for all reactions. Glucose tablets relieve symptoms faster than anything else and can be precisely measured to prevent overtreatment. Glucose or dextrose tablets can be obtained from many pharmacies and from most of the mail order diabetes supply stores.

- If glucose tablets aren't available, reduce the amount of carbohydrate that is used. For most reactions, 15 grams of fast-acting carbohydrate will bring the low blood sugar quickly back to normal. Fifteen grams is the equivalent of a cup of milk and one square graham cracker, or two-thirds of a banana, or 4 to 5 ounces of a regular soda. Have 15 grams and, in 20 minutes when brain function has returned, retest your blood sugar. Then consider if you really need more carbohydrate.

- If you are unable to stop yourself from overeating, calculate the total amount of carbohydrate you have eaten, and subtract the amount needed to cover your reaction. Cover most of the extra carbohydrate **above what you needed to treat your reaction** with a carbohydrate bolus.

- If you have frequent blood sugars below 70 mg/dl, review your basal and bolus settings to determine where this excess insulin is coming from. If uncertain about how to change your insulin, contact your physician/health care team immediately.

VARIABLE LIFESTYLE

People are usually aware of how consistent their lifestyle is. Whether or not one eats and sleeps at regular times and gets exercise on a regular schedule is easy to recognize. Whether or not work or school schedules are consistent is also important to recognize.

In determining basal rates and boluses, it helps to have a consistent lifestyle. If you have an irregular lifestyle and variable blood sugars are occurring, create as stable a lifestyle as you can to sort out the causes. Then, if necessary, go back to your previous schedule, using caution.

PATTERN:

The lack of a pattern is the pattern.

WHAT TO DO:

- Carefully test and chart your blood sugars seven times a day, together with accompanying narrative regarding stress, exercise periods, general health, etc.

- Eat meals with the same amount of carbohydrate and at the same time of day for awhile.

- Exercise regularly and consistently. Note whether the type, amount or timing of exercise has variable effects on your blood sugars.

- Working the overnight shift is usually not a great problem, especially if the weekend schedule does not vary greatly from the weekday schedule.

- If you work a rotating shift, it may be worthwhile staying on a single shift until the pump is correctly set. Talk with your employer to see if this can be done. If blood sugar control is poor and you work a rotating shift, seek the help of your physician/ health care team to sort out this situation.

CARBOHYDRATE PROBLEMS

One of the most critical elements for controlling blood sugars is to match carbohydrate intake to insulin doses. The most frequent cause for variable blood sugars is some problem related to the matchup between carbohydrates and the meal bolus. We'll discuss four areas where problems with carbohydrates can occur.

1. MEASUREMENT ERRORS

Good blood sugar control is difficult if you are not accurately measuring carbohydrates. When the amount of carbohydrate in a meal is unknown, it's impossible to give an accurate carbohydrate bolus. Problems can arise from inexperience in measuring carbohydrates, from frequently eating out where carbohydrate quantities must be estimated, or from simply not measuring.

PATTERN:

If your basal rate tests were good, but your blood sugars vary when you eat, consider that the problem may be in measuring carbohydrates. On your Advanced Workshop Charts, look for a high or low blood sugar related to a particular meal, especially if the meal was eaten at a restaurant or friend's house, or if you haven't had this meal before.

Let's say you need 1 unit of Regular for each 10 grams of carbohydrate. Suppose you usually eat 70 grams of carbohydrate for dinner and have great blood sugars with a 7 unit bolus. But one evening you have "70 grams" covered with a 7 unit bolus and your blood sugar rises. Be suspicious that you miscalculated the carbohydrate in that meal.

WHAT TO DO:

- If you suspect inaccurate measurement is a problem, review how to measure carbohydrates with your nutritionist or physician/health care team.

- If you eat out often, try eating a favorite meal at the same restaurant until you can cover it well with a bolus. On each occasion, record how many grams of carbohydrate you estimate the meal contains and how many units of insulin you took to cover it. It will become obvious after a few tries how many units you need for that meal. This carbohydrate bolus will then give you a good estimate for the actual number of grams of carbohydrate in the meal. Some of the books listed in Chapter 6 are very handy for eating out. They give a comprehensive list of foods found in different types of restaurants and the number of grams of carbohydrate they contain.

- Take your gram scale and the Carbohydrate Index in Appendix A with you to the restaurant. Don't worry. People do strange things in restaurants. Pretend you are a government inspector or food critic. Some self-consciousness will be more than offset by your improved control and the extra service you receive from the waiter.

2. VARIATIONS IN MEAL SIZE AND TIMING

Although pumping is the best method for having variety in your life, variations in the size and timing of meals can make stable blood sugars hard to achieve, especially if your Carbohydrate Boluses have never been tested, or the testing was inconsistent due to a free-form lifestyle.

PATTERN:

Here the pattern is the lack of pattern, with only random day-to-day variation. This variation is easy to spot on your charts. Blood sugars will rise and fall, but more importantly **the timing of meals and the carbohydrate in them will vary significantly from one day to the next**.

WHAT TO DO:

Allow yourself the chance to stabilize. It helps to live life more routinely for a few weeks as you first go on your pump or if your blood sugar control has been poor. Give yourself a period in your life when you avoid foods high in sugar and fat, and eat the same amounts of carbohydrates at set times. Set up your pump to this consistency, and once you're well-controlled, begin reintroducing variety into your life. You'll find you can handle the changes you want much easier from a stable base of blood sugars.

3. Variations in the Glycemic Index

As noted in Chapter 6, not all carbohydrates are equal. Fifty grams of carbohydrate from ice cream can have a totally different effect on your blood sugar than fifty grams from a bowl of Cornflakes®. Although you're eating the same amount of carbohydrate, you'll find that your blood sugar rises higher and faster when you have the Cornflakes®.

When nutritionists realized that different carbohydrates can affect blood sugars differently, they attempted to quantify these differences by developing a glycemic index. A single glycemic index that everyone agrees on cannot be developed due to variations in how individuals respond to the same food. A variety of glycemic indexes exists, each providing a rough guide to how different foods will affect your blood sugar. Appendix B gives the glycemic indexes for various foods adapted from a review of several studies done by David Jenkins and others (*Diabetes Care* 11: 149-159, 1988).

Pattern:

Offensive foods will show up on your postmeal blood sugar readings. If you start with an 82, shoot up to 317 two hours later, and are back down to 123 before the next meal, you have covered your carbohydrate with the correct bolus. However, you either did not take your insulin soon enough before the meal or you ate a carbohydrate with a high glycemic index.

What To Do:

- Refer to the Glycemic Index in Appendix B. Check the foods you are eating against those listed. If your foods have a high rating, switch to foods that have a lower rating.

- Avoid foods with a high glycemic rating. If you eat them, try taking your meal bolus earlier than usual to offset this faster acting carbohydrate.

- Shift to different types or brands of foods. Instead of a wheat or corn-based cereal, try one made from oats or rice, such as Cheerios®, or one with more fiber, such as All Bran® or Shredded Wheat and Bran®. Instead of a banana, try strawberries. Instead of white rice, try brown rice.

4. Unusual Food Effects

Some foods have unexpected effects on the blood sugar. Candies sweetened with sorbitol may send blood sugars higher than expected. Peanuts and pretzels often raise blood sugars more than expected. Chinese foods and pizza are renowned for their ability to raise blood sugars.

Occasionally, an individual will have a unique response to a food. One pumper had frequent, high blood sugars that were unexplainable until she noticed that they always occurred several hours after meals that contained two or more ounces of cheese. Research has shown that pizza raises blood sugars higher than the carbohydrate content suggests it should,[80] confirming the experience many people have had with it. Some have noted that pizza that is lower in fat, such as a vegetarian one, does not raise the blood sugar as high.

PATTERN:

Look for a consistent rise in your blood sugar when you eat a particular food.

WHAT TO DO:

- Write down all the foods you eat on your charts, not just the carbohydrates.

- If you suspect a particular food affects your blood sugar, record your blood sugar readings when you eat it. Compare these readings to other meals with similar amounts of carbohydrate to see if there's a difference. If you are suspicious of a food that is low in carbohydrate such as cheese or meat, leave it out or reduce it in quantity to see what effect it is having. If you see a pattern of rising blood sugars after eating a suspected food, eliminate it from your meals or reduce the amount you eat.

- If you suspect blood sugar variability because of your foods, you may need the assistance of your physician or nutritionist to sort it out. Be sure to seek their advice if you suspect you have a food-related problem, but are unable to determine its source.

STRESS

Stress is a natural part of being human. Without stress, we would not have the challenges that offer growth, the conflicts that pinpoint areas of our personality in need of change, nor the losses from which to gather strength. But stress can be overwhelming at times. Difficult times may be an extended illness, the death of a family member or friend, or a problematic work situation or relationship. The combination of several factors may occur at one time.

Stress interferes with blood sugar control in several ways. When stressful events occur, it is difficult to continue normal patterns of living. Eating, sleeping and exercise may all be altered. Sleep may be lost during periods of stress, exercise and other calming activities may be put aside, and fast foods high in sugar and fat may be eaten more often. Difficulties in controlling blood sugars during stress are often related to the difficulty in maintaining a sense of order in daily life.

Stress also interferes with blood sugar control through an excessive release of stress hormones. Fight or flight hormones help us remain alert and active during stress. Unfortunately, they also interfere with insulin's action, and cause extra glucose to be produced and released into the blood. This results in higher blood sugars than usual and the need for more insulin.

Emotions and blood sugars are interrelated. During emotional periods, blood sugars usually rise. High blood sugars cause more stress hormones to be released, which then magnify emotional reactions. Elevated blood sugars can also cause changes within brain cells that promote depression and irritability. The result is an impaired ability to deal with the stress at hand.

122

Stress and frustration can also result from the challenge of caring for your diabetes. During your first attempts at controlling blood sugars, frustration from the seeming magnitude of the job can set in. Ongoing attempts at control can be stressful, especially when results are slow to be seen.

PATTERN:

Generally, very little pattern exists. Some stress, especially that related to work, will decrease on weekends or during vacations. If you feel like a totally different person when you have had a few days off, or you find your blood sugars are much easier to control at these times, consider carefully how much stress you may be under. Others often see the extent of our stress before we do and their comments may be the first indication of our own level of stress.

WHAT TO DO:

- Practice good eating habits all the time. If you avoid candy bars when life is going well, you are less likely to pick up a candy bar when stress hits.

- Test your blood sugars. With stress, testing and exercise are often the first things dropped from your lifestyle. Testing makes normal blood sugars possible and with normal blood sugars, brain function improves and stress hormone levels are lower. Whatever the source of stress, it can be handled better when in good control.

- Take time daily to exercise, especially when stressed. A walk can do wonders. Exercise releases endorphins in the brain to help you feel better and handle stress better.

- Be aware that the demands of blood glucose monitoring, counting carbohydrates, and blood glucose regulation can be overwhelming at times. Take a break from these routines when you need one. Determine how much time off you need to clear your mind. Take the time needed, and come back to your monitoring with new vigor.

- If you feel frustrated by your blood sugar readings or doubt that you can make any sense out of your Advanced Workshop Charts, seek the help of someone who does not share your frustration. Talk with your physician for help or for a referral to someone who specializes in blood sugar control.

- How you respond to stress is largely a learned process. If you note frequent high blood sugars following job pressure, arguments, or bad news, seek the advice of a specialist in how to better handle your responses. Stress management classes are offered by community colleges and by many employers.

- Talk. Stress is always worse when carried alone. Share your feelings, worries, guilt and pain with others. No burden is too great to share with others.

"Eloquence is logic on fire."

Lyman Beecher

PUMPING INSULIN

CELLULAR FRONTIERS:
PREVENTING AND REVERSING COMPLICATIONS

20

Everyone dreads complications from diabetes, but do they have to occur? In this chapter we'll describe some of the ways in which damage occurs and discuss ways to minimize the damage. In the Diabetes Control and Complications Trial a linear relationship (depicted by the solid line in Fig. 20.1) was found between blood sugar control, measured by the HbA1c level, and risks for eye and kidney disease. That is, for every increase in average blood sugar level, eye and kidney complications are more likely. This is believed to be true as well for other complications.

High blood sugars are **far more likely to lead to complications.** No matter what else is said, this rule remains in effect. The best way to stay healthy is **always keep your blood sugars as normal as possible.** Keeping blood sugar levels in the normal range, however, isn't possible for everyone. A person may live alone, drive a truck, or have erratic physical demands at work and need to keep blood sugars higher to guarantee that no serious low blood sugars occur.

But do high blood sugars always mean complications? Note again the **solid diagonal line** in Figure 20.1, representing an average risk for physical damage found in people with diabetes over a wide range of HbA1c values.

Half of those with diabetes are above the diagonal line and have a greater than average risk for complications. The other half fall below the line where complications are fewer. And some people are far to the right and near the bottom.

Figure 20.1 Can The Risk For Complications Be Lowered?

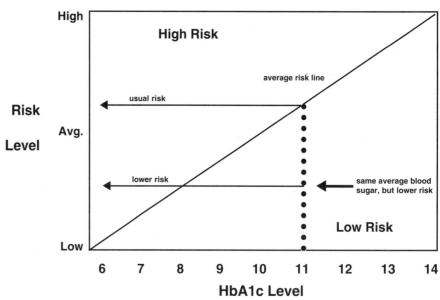

That is, for the same average blood sugar and duration of diabetes, these people have **less risk of physical damage**. For example, even though a person in this group runs a HbA1c of 11%, for some reason he has a relatively low risk for complications. Of course, everyone wants to be in a lower risk group.

Something is different about these people. It could be their genes, but multiple research studies show only weak relationships between genetic makeup and the risks for complications. Not to be ignored, but not an overwhelming player. Other protective factors appear to be involved.

What are these protective factors and, more importantly, can any of them be controlled so you can place yourself in the safer (lower) regions of Figure 20.1 regardless of your blood sugar control? Some strategies are simple. Keeping the blood pressure normal is smart. Regular aerobic and strength-training exercises are direct deposits into a longevity account. (They also make daily life more fun and keep us physically independent as we age.) Not smoking is a windfall. (Fortunately, fewer than 1 in 9 of those with Type I diabetes and 1 in 6 of those with Type II diabetes smoke.) Less fat in the diet along with a higher percentage of essential fatty acids from seeds and fish helps. Five servings of vegetables and fruits beats simply eating an apple a day. A body weight near ideal keeps the mortician's thumbs twiddling, as does reducing stress and improving our reactions to stressful events.

The health advantage of some of these interventions is significant. For instance, in the MR FIT study of risk factors in over 340,000 American men, those with lower systolic blood pressures and cholesterol levels had much lower death rates.[81] Over 5,000 of these men reported taking medications for diabetes. In this subgroup with diabetes, the death rate was between 155 and 242 deaths per 10,000 person-years in those whose systolic blood pressure was above 160 mm of mercury, but fewer than 66 deaths per 10,000 person-years when the blood pressure was below 140 mm. If the blood pressure is lowered with medicines that do not themselves cause excess deaths, it is highly likely that a person who has high blood pressure will live longer when their blood pressure is lowered.

Lowering the cholesterol level may have benefits as well. In this same study when those who had a cholesterol over 260 mg/dl were compared to those with a level below 180, the death rate fell from about 130 per 10,000 person-years to around 62. This assumes, of course, that it's actually the cholesterol creating the excess mortality, and that a particular cholesterol therapy or medication does not itself have negative effects.

Strategies like these are widely accepted, but other mechanisms are also at work. Diabetes creates a high blood sugar environment in which aging is accelerated,[82] and in which heart disease, cataracts and other age-related problems occur at an earlier age. At the root of complications, cellular mechanisms operate. By understanding these mechanisms, interventions to prevent complications can be better planned and have greater results. Cell mechanics, though still a young science, is beginning to bear fruit. Benefits to health and longevity can happen if we follow health-enhancing strategies, and we learn how to enhance cellular mechanisms to slow aging and prevent cell damage in diabetes.

It is useful to examine research studies and experimental results that point to solutions to the ongoing problem of complications. Keep in mind that other mechanisms believed to be involved are not discussed in this short chapter. Areas that are discussed include:

- pseudohypoxia,
- protein glycosylation,
- oxidation,
- myoinositol and ATP imbalances, and
- lipid and clotting abnormalities.

As we discuss different mechanisms, realize that no one of them is totally responsible. They may all play a role. The pace of developments as researchers sort out the importance of each one has been slow and the reason is simple: complications are that---complicated. Don't expect any magic bullets. Instead, look for interventions suggested by research that you can take within your own life to make you a healthier person.

PSEUDOHYPOXIA

The theory of pseudohypoxia was introduced in June, 1993, at the American Diabetes Association Conference in Las Vegas. The theory represents international collaboration between researchers in St. Louis, Missouri; Nagoya, Japan; Aarhus, Denmark; and Antwerp, Belguim.[83] Pseudohypoxia helps explain many of the observed effects of diabetes, and better, it lays out **several ways in which damage from high blood sugars might be stopped or lessened.**

At the ADA Conference, Ronald Tilton, Ph.D., of Washington University School of Medicine explained pseudohypoxia. In simple terms, this theory holds that exposure to high blood sugar for periods longer than four or five hours causes blood vessels to dilate and blood flow to increase. These changes are very similar to what happens when cells lack oxygen. Although oxygen **is not lacking**, the metabolism of the cells changes **as if oxygen deprivation exists**, hence the name. If cells act as though they are not getting oxygen, this can have major impact on situations like angina and heart disease. It has direct relevance to nerves which depend on an oxygen supply through blood vessels that are smaller in diameter than a red blood cell, and to proliferative retinopathy where abnormal blood vessel growth is thought to occur as a result of an oxygen deficit.

Pseudohypoxia expands on the theory of the aldose reductase pathway (see pages 133 and 134) as a mechanism for damage. Aldose reductase has its critics,[84, 85] but, as noted by Dr. Tilton and his associates, many of the changes suggested by the pseudohypoxia theory have been tested and appear to have merit. Some of the excess glucose in high blood sugars is converted to sorbitol, and then, in a second step, the sorbitol is converted to fructose or fruit sugar. High fructose levels in the body are found with poorly controlled diabetes. Due to the increased conversion of sorbitol to fructose in this second step, there is a drop in levels of NAD+, a molecule that stores and transports energy in cells. This causes cells to develop a lower electrical charge, much like a weak battery in a toy.

A series of destructive changes ensues: more dilation of blood vessels, increased blood flow (called microvascular hypertension), excess oxidation and free radical production, leaky blood vessels, loss of sodium-potassium ATPase activity (linked to high blood pressure, kidney disease, insulin resistance, and other problems), accumulation of fructose (which leads to excess protein glycosylation, described below), gradual hardening of blood vessels and loss of blood flow, and weakening of the heart. Fortunately, almost all of these damage mechanisms have potential for drug and biochemical interventions that may block their effects.

PROTEIN GLYCOSYLATION

When blood sugars are normal, a few glucose molecules will attach themselves to nearby proteins. But as blood sugars rise, **more glucose attaches to more proteins**. A protein which has glucose attached to it, called a glycosylated protein, is damaged. In an environment of high blood sugars, more of these damaged proteins are found. Since proteins create structures and enzymes throughout the body, this type of damage becomes widespread. A few protein-rich structures where damage may occur are the lens of the eye, skin, tendons, cartilage, cell membranes and blood vessel walls.

Other proteins act as enzymes which perform complex biochemical processes. Both enzymes and structural proteins need precise structures to do their work. Unfortunately, **glycosylation of proteins damages these structures**.[86] As glycosylated proteins accumulate, structures become weaker and enzymes perform less work.

Protein glycosylation is believed to contribute to nerve damage,[87] eye damage,[88] kidney damage, arthritis, DNA damage, cataracts, high blood pressure and blood vessel damage. Arthritis and joint problems are more common with diabetes.[89] The link between high blood sugars and joint problems is partly due to glycosylation of collagen, a structural protein in joints. Glycosylation roughens and thickens tendons and joint surfaces. Another cause for joint problems may be the excess levels of superoxide free radicals found in poorly controlled diabetes.[90] (See Figure 20.3 on page 132.) Superoxide radicals target collagen for damage and superoxide radicals are created **at much faster rates by proteins which are glycosylated**.

Glucose has even been shown to glycosylate DNA in bacteria and presumably does the same in humans.[86] The significance of this is unknown, although damage to mitochondrial DNA is one of the suspected causes of aging[91] and also of Type I diabetes itself.[92]

Cataracts are another byproduct of protein glycosylation. The lens at the front of the eye allows us to see the world. About 98% of the dry weight of the lens is made of proteins that are straight and arranged to let light pass through, much like an open venetian blind. These structural proteins can become damaged, either by oxidizing radiation found in sunlight (which is why sunglasses and antioxidants are used to prevent cataracts), or by glycosylation. On average, cataracts occur 10 to 15 years earlier in people with poorly-controlled diabetes. Another factor that doubles the risk of cataracts is smoking, partly from the increased oxidation created by toxic smoke.

Another change in body structures found with poor control is the development of thickened basement membranes. Normal basement membrane is a thin, supporting matrix of protein found in small blood vessel walls, muscles, kidneys and eyes. With high blood sugars, these membranes thicken partly as a result of excess glycosylation. They become stiff and allow large proteins to leak through. Thicker blood vessel walls raise the blood pressure. Thickening of basement membranes can be reversed by bringing the blood sugars under better control.

Protein glycosylation has been used to develop lab tests that measure long term blood sugar control. One test is the HbA1c or glycosylated hemoglobin test. Hemoglobin is a protein, so this test is actually a glycosylated protein test. The more glucose in the blood, the more that attaches to hemoglobin. The HbA1c measures the percentage of the protein hemoglobin in the body which has glucose attached to it.

Another test, called the fructosamine test, measures how much glucose is attached to a wider range of proteins, not just to the hemoglobin that carries oxygen. The fructosamine and HbA1c tests provide a way to measure blood sugar control over the previous 3 and 8 weeks respectively. **They also provide a picture of the amount of internal protein damage that has been occurring.**

Glycosylation of proteins is bad enough. However, in a process called the Maillard reaction, two glycosylated proteins that are close to each other become cross-linked to form **permanently** damaged structures called **Advanced Glycosylation Endproducts or AGEs**. AGEs, as the name implies, are thought to contribute to the accelerated aging found in a high blood sugar environment.

AGE-LDL (that's LDL or "bad" cholesterol with AGE in its protein structure) **is found at extremely high levels in people who have both diabetes and kidney disease**. In one study, a nondiabetic control group had 109 units of AGE per milligram of lipid (fat), but in those with diabetes and advanced kidney disease 3,270 units were present, **30 times normal levels**.[93] Kidney disease is associated with higher rates of oxidation and glycosylation of proteins, leading to this excess formation of AGEs.

AGEs, in turn, prevent cells lining the blood vessels from forming nitric oxide. Nitric oxide allows blood vessels to relax and also prevents an abnormal proliferation of cells within the blood vessel.[94] This proliferation of cells and the presence of abnormal protein structures with blood vessels and kidney cells are believed to be major contributors to kidney disease and to the much higher risk for heart disease that accompanies kidney disease.[95] When AGEs are found in myelin, the protective outer coating of nerves, these AGEs are nine times as likely to cause an attack by the immune system.[87] This immune system attack on abnormal nerve structures is believed to be one of the causes for nerve damage.

Dr. Michael Brownlee, mentioned in Chapter 3, is working with a research drug called aminoguanidine to see if the glycosylation leading to permanently damaged AGEs can be stopped. But concern in the use of aminoguanidine is warranted because it can lead to high histamine levels in a few susceptible individuals.[40] Excessive histamine can create a severe medical emergency in these individuals. In less toxic amounts it can increase leakage of proteins through blood vessels, which might worsen complications like macular edema or kidney disease.

Another intervention being considered to decrease glycosylation is the use of D-lysine, a biologically inactive form of the amino acid lysine. Lysine is a primary target for glycosylation in proteins. By giving D-lysine to animals, researchers have been able to decrease glycosylation.[96] No studies have been done in humans and the long-term effects of this treatment are unknown. Watch for developments regarding these and other drugs that are designed to stop glycosylation.

In an interesting development, researchers at the University of South Carolina showed that glycosylation of proteins is a reversible process. But once a glycosylated protein becomes oxidized, it is then able to form the permanently cross-linked AGEs. This places the oxidation process (discussed next) in a critical role, because much more is known about how to prevent oxidation than glycosylation. These researchers went on to say, "It has always been puzzling that...there are patients in poor glycemic control who appear resistant to complications....The solution to this riddle may lie in the relationship between glycation and oxidation and differences in oxidative stress among diabetes patients."[97]

OXIDATION

A destructive process that everyone faces, more oxidation occurs when blood sugars are high. Oxygen allows life and is essential for the conversion of fuels like glucose and fat into energy, but it also causes rust, the oxidation of iron. Some 2% of the oxygen used by the body generates unwanted, highly-reactive free radicals, which do not follow the normal rules of metabolism but creates "rust" in the body. Additional free radicals are also generated in harmful environments like smoking, smog and solar radiation.

The molecules from which we're made require stability, but they are stable only when they contain **paired** orbiting electrons. Free radicals contain **an unpaired electron**. With an unpaired electron, molecules become **unstable** until they give this unpaired electron to a neighboring molecule, or steal one from another molecule. This electron imbalance **creates a chain-reaction of destructive molecular dominoes**. Molecules with an unpaired electron become temporary free radicals, causing damage and fragmentation in random fashion. Random destruction continues until the electron is captured by a system of defenses known as antioxidants.

Free radicals destroy cell structures. Any fatty acid, protein, or enzyme which comes in contact with a free radical may have its structure crippled or severed. Bruce N. Ames of the University of California at Berkeley estimates that the DNA within each human cell takes 10,000 direct hits from free radicals each day. Free radicals often start the process of protein cross-linking that generates Advanced Glycosylation Endproducts (AGEs) mentioned in the last section. Free radicals are suspected of contributing to cancer and aging,[98] and of being a factor in several types of brain damage, including that caused by very severe insulin reactions.[99, 100] (Luckily, insulin reactions this severe are very rare.)

128

Some of this damage can be repaired by built-in mechanisms cells have for repairing oxidative damage. However, as cells spend more time on these repairs **they spend less time on processes related to health**. An individual's ability to handle free radicals is thought to play a major role in health and lifespan.

ANTIOXIDANTS

Antioxidants disarm free radicals, but what are they? Antioxidants are a varied group of vitamins and mineral-containing enzymes. The most widely known are vitamins C, E and beta carotene; others include superoxide dismutase, quercitin, glutathione, selenium, ginko biloba and lipoic acid. They stop destruction by balancing the unpaired electron in a free radical. After balancing an unpaired electron, an antioxidant remains relatively stable and the disarmed free radical is no longer harmful.

Antioxidants perform their role in different ways in different parts of the body. Vitamin C, for instance, is water soluble and deactivates free radicals in the cytoplasm, the water-based fluid inside the cell. A cell deficiency of vitamin C, called **intracellular scurvy**, is believed to contribute to the blood vessel damage found in diabetes.[101]

Other antioxidants, like vitamin E and beta carotene, are fat soluble and protect fat-containing cell membranes and cholesterol in the blood. Superoxide dismutase or SOD, another antioxidant, converts the superoxide free radical (an oxygen molecule with a spare electron that likes to damage collagen) into hydrogen peroxide. Hydrogen peroxide is then converted into harmless water and oxygen by the antioxidants glutathione peroxidase and catalase.

People with diabetes have long been recognized as subject to excess oxidation[102, 103] and are known to have low levels of protective antioxidants.[104, 105] Disturbances of antioxidants and other vitamins have been well-documented in diabetes.[106, 107] For example, the antioxidant vitamin C is low in diabetes despite adequate intake of this vitamin in the diet.[108]

Several studies done in the general population show how important antioxidant levels are. Serum vitamin E has been shown to have a clear inverse relationship to the incidence of angina. A low level of serum vitamin E was a better predictor of this disease than serum cholesterol, hypertension or smoking in one population-based study.[109] In another major study of 16 different European populations, Swiss researchers found that "vitamin E is the most important factor to explain cross-cultural differences in ischemic heart disease mortality."[110]

A bioflavanoid antioxidant called quercitin, found mainly in tea and apples, was monitored in another study. In this study of 805 men over the age of 65, higher dietary quercitin was associated with a **27% lower risk of dying**. Cardiac mortality, in particular, dropped by 50%, probably due to the ability of flavanoids to inhibit LDL oxidation and to their protective effect in sequestering already-oxidized LDL.[111] In a double-blind study, beta carotene or a placebo was used in 333 physicians. Those in the beta carotene group had a **44% reduction in major coronary events**.[112]

Harvard epidemiologists looked at vitamin E intake in nearly 40,000 physicians and in 87,000 nurses over periods of 4 years and 8 years respectively. A strong association was found between vitamin E intake and less risk for heart disease. Men who took at least 100 units of vitamin E a day were **37% less likely to have heart disease**.[113] In this study, beta carotene intake also appeared to protect those who smoked cigarettes. Women who took vitamin E for 2 years or more were **41% less likely** to suffer from heart disease.[114]

Another large study, called NHANES I, followed more than 11,000 United States adults between the years 1971 and 1984. UCLA researchers, led by Dr. James Enstrom, looked at this data and found that men who had higher vitamin C intake from both diet and supplements had a **35% lower death rate**.[115] Women in this study did not fare as well, managing only a 10% reduction in mortality, possibly due to a lower risk for heart disease where most of the benefit for men was seen. Cancer deaths were 22% lower in men and 14% lower in women.

It should be noted that not every study of vitamin C has found this reduction in mortality. The Harvard study just quoted found no association between vitamin C intake and protection from heart disease. And the effects of using large doses of antioxidants over long periods of time has not been thoroughly studied, although we can assume that anything becomes toxic when too much of it is taken. But the general trend is for lower rates of heart disease, cancer and death in the great majority of studies on antioxidant intake.

Taking antioxidant supplements, like vitamin C and vitamin E, appear to help counteract free radical damage, but there are some limits. After balancing an electron with a free radical and disarming it, an antioxidant has to **have its own electrons restored to a paired state** before it can return to its work as an antioxidant. When vitamins C and E pick up a free radical, **they themselves become weak free radical generators!** For instance, when vitamin C or ascorbic acid balances the extra electron in a free radical it becomes dihydroascorbate or DHA. DHA levels are found to be high in diabetes. DHA causes unwanted AGEs to form and is believed to be a major factor in creating cataracts in diabetes.[116]

Only after these vitamins are cleansed in a process involving glutathione do they again become safe and return to their role as protectors. Glutathione takes a free radical from DHA and places the cleansed vitamin C back into action. To play its protective role, glutathione itself has to be recycled by the enzyme glutathione peroxidase. Unfortunately, the activity of glutathione peroxidase is low in diabetes.[117] This causes glutathione levels to drop and allows damaging forms of vitamins C and E to accumulate.

Glutathione peroxidase is most active and will best perform its role in defending the body **when blood sugars are normal**. In people who do not have diabetes, glutathione has been increased by taking a vitamin C supplement.[118] In those with diabetes, vitamin E has been shown to lower the amount of "bad" glutathione by 50% with no change in the blood sugar level.[119] Another antioxidant, the trace mineral selenium, also appears to increase glutathione levels. It appears hopeful, paticularly given the number of studies showing that antioxidants protect against heart disease, cataracts and other diabetes-related complications, that these complications can be reduced by diets high in antioxidants and by adding antioxidant supplements.

Studies like these led the respected U. C. Berkeley epidemiologist Gladys Block, M.D. to observe, *"In the United States, plasma ascorbate levels are disturbingly low in major segments of the population, reflecting equally disturbingly low intake. The results of Enstom et al indicate that increased attention should be given not only to dietary sources of these nutrients, but also to the possible benefits of vitamin supplements."*[120] Dr. Block has also surveyed over a hundred research studies that have looked at the relationship between antioxidant intake and cancer. In her survey, she found 120 of these 130 studies showed less risk for cancer when people had a higher intake of various antioxidants[121] (see also the box on page 132).

ARE ANTIOXIDANTS PROTECTIVE?

The two processes of protein glycosylation and oxidation by free radicals are intertwined in a cycle of damage and destruction. In the test tube, glycosylated proteins can produce **50 times** as many superoxide radicals as non-glycosylated proteins.[122] The reverse is also true: **more oxidation causes more glycosylation of proteins!** The good news is that antioxidants counter the destructive processes of both oxidation and glycosylation. In one study of 12 people without diabetes who took 1000 mg of the antioxidant vitamin C daily for 3 months to curtail oxidation, researchers found that their glycosylated hemoglobin (HbA1c) was lowered by 18%, and another

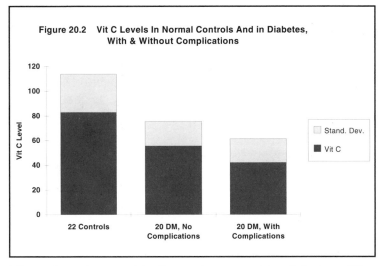

Figure 20.2   Vit C Levels In Normal Controls And in Diabetes,
With & Without Complications

protein, albumin, had 33% less glucose attached to it.[123] (Yes, this may help lower your HbA1c test, and no, it is not cheating.) In other studies, vitamin E was shown to lower blood sugar levels[124] and to lower HbA1c levels in people with Type II diabetes.[125] By lessening glycosylation, antioxidants keep proteins in better shape, enzymes more active, and lessen the risk for excess oxidation from glycosylated proteins.

Diabetes is characterized by faster aging. Both oxidation[98] and glycosylation[82] are thought to contribute to aging, and both are increased in diabetes. Glucose will itself create free radicals that damage protein structures in a process called autoglycosylation.[126]

As noted above, low levels of antioxidants like vitamin C, vitamin E, and glutathione are found in most studies of diabetes.[127] In one study, blood vitamin C levels were measured in 22 people without diabetes, in 20 people with diabetes who had no complications, and in 20 people with diabetes who had complications. Figure 20.2 shows the marked drop in the level of vitamin C in diabetes and the even greater decrease when complications are present.[128]

In another study, vitamin C levels were found to be lower in a group of elderly people with diabetes, especially in those who had eye damage.[129] Authors of this study proposed that vitamin C becomes a "sacrificial lamb" to the excess oxidation occurring in retinopathy, and that this drop in vitamin C levels shows the excessive oxidative stress placed on cells.

Besides the hampered recycling of vitamin C due to low glutathione levels, vitamin C is also lost because it competes with glucose for transport. The structures of vitamin C and glucose are almost identical, so they use many of the same pathways for transport. When blood sugar levels are high, less vitamin C is transported into cells where it becomes concentrated at 25 to 80 times the level found in the blood. Vitamin C is also consumed in an environment of increased oxidation found with high levels of glycosylated proteins.

The antioxidant vitamin E is needed by platelets to stop them from producing the clotting factor thromboxane. Platelets travel in the blood and provide the clotting factors needed to repair blood vessels, but when thromboxane levels are too high, excess clotting occurs that can damage both large and small blood vessels. Small blood vessel or microvascular damage is linked to eye, nerve and kidney complications. In a sudy of 16 people without diabetes, vitamin E levels were measured at 295 ng per 10^9 platelets, while in 16 people who had Type I diabetes levels of vitamin E were only 170 ng per 10^9 platelets.[130] In a Vienna, Austria study, supplements containing vitamin E were shown to lower the excess production of thromboxane in 22 Type I diabetics.[131]

Vitamin E also appears to protect against glycosylation. In a study of rats, a non-diabetic control group was compared to two groups with diabetes. One diabetic group was given vitamin E and one was not. The HbA1c level in the nondiabetic control group was 2.6% compared to 7.7% in the rats with diabetes who did not get vitamin E. But the rats with diabetes given vitamin E had a level of only 5.5%, despite blood sugars as high as the other diabetes group.[132]

One antioxidant, an enzyme called superoxide dismutase or SOD, protects the body by counteracting the superoxide free radical. SOD is damaged and less active once it becomes glycosylated by high blood sugars.[133] Low levels of SOD are found along with high levels of superoxide radicals in environments with high blood sugars[90, 134] or high triglyceride levels.[135]

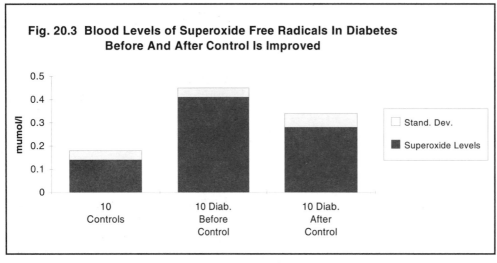

Fig. 20.3 Blood Levels of Superoxide Free Radicals In Diabetes Before And After Control Is Improved

As early as 1980, it was known that high blood sugar levels caused an excess production of superoxide radicals.[136] Researchers checked the blood for damaging superoxide radicals in 10 people with diabetes and in 10 people without diabetes and found far higher levels in those who had diabetes.[90] Superoxide levels were then remeasured after blood sugar control was improved. Figure 20.3 shows the results: better blood sugar control caused a **marked drop in how many superoxide radicals were produced**.

Antioxidants, like vitamin E and superoxide dismutase, are present at higher levels in the healthy retina than in most other tissues, suggesting they are important in protecting the eyes. Our ability to see is a result of the retina's ability to sense light, color and shape via neurons transmitting this information to the brain. One test of eye health, called an electroretinogram or ERG, involves shining light onto the retina and then measuring the speed and strength of electrical messages sent to the brain. The ERG test gives early warning of damage to the retina or its associated nerves. In diabetic rats, the ERG amplitude was reduced by 60% after only 2 months of exposure to high blood sugars. However, another group of diabetic rats treated with the herbal antioxidant ginko biloba were found to have significantly better retina function at the end of two months.[137]

Whether the higher production of free radicals and lower protection from antioxidants in diabetes actually cause diabetic complications is still not known. It could be that these lowered antioxidant levels are only a minor factor in the damage found with high blood sugars. It seems clear, however, that antioxidants are critical to protecting cells and when their levels are low, more oxidative damage and more glycosylation of proteins will occur. **This situation seems highly likely to increase damage associated with complications and to compromise health.**

Some research is beginning to appear regarding the use of antioxidants

After more than 40 years of research, so little risk has been found and the potential benefits are so great that the editorial board of the Berkeley Wellness Letter recommends an antioxidant supplement for all healthy adults.[127] They recommend an intake of 10,000 to 25,000 units of beta carotene, 250 to 500 mg of vitamin C, and 200 to 800 units of vitamin E.

"Supplements of beta carotene and Vitamin E seem to have no significant side effects, even in large amounts. Up to 1,000 milligrams of vitamin C a day also produces no ill effects." according to the nationally respected Berkeley Wellness Letter. (October, 1991) (Excess beta carotene can cause the skin to turn orange in a condition called carotinemia.)

A vitamin supplement specifically designed for diabetes has been developed by pharmacist R. Keith Campbell, Associate Dean of Pharmacy at Washington State University. Keith has diabetes and is nationally recognized for his diabetes work. This supplement has excellent antioxidant levels, as well as B vitamins and minerals. Information may be obtained from Jordan Medical Enterprises, Inc. in Garden Grove, California at 1-800-541-1193

132

to prevent complications. German researchers tried various antioxidants (vitamin E, selenium and lipoic acid) in 80 patients with diabetes who had advanced diabetes complications. In the treated groups, the researchers found significantly less oxidative damage and less leakage of microalbumin through the kidneys. They also measured significant improvements in peripheral nerve damage. The authors of this study proposed that treatment with antioxidants may lead to a lower risk of complications.[139]

AR, SDH, MYOINOSITOL AND ATP

Another mechanism by which complications develop and a key step in the pseudohypoxia theory involves the funnelling of excess glucose into the byproducts sorbitol and fructose. Both byproducts are found at high levels with poor control. Their buildup depends on high blood sugars and involves two enzymes: aldose reductase (AR) and sorbitol dehydrogenase (SDH). AR converts glucose to sorbitol and SDH converts sorbitol to fructose.

Overactivity of the enzyme SDH wastes energy stored as NAD+ as the enzyme creates fructose from excess sorbitol. NAD+ is used to drive many of the enzymes needed for health. When less NAD+ is available, the enzymes it drives become less active. One result of this is the accumulation of lactic acid--a substance familiar to exhausted athletes. Another is the loss of the protective antioxidant glutathione.

Sorbitol also competes with myoinositol for entry in cells, causing myoinositol levels to drop. Myoinositol is a compound that helps to form ATP, which like NAD+ acts as a "battery" within the cell to store energy. As myoinositol levels drop, the cells of someone with diabetes lose as much as 30% of their energy stored in the form of ATP. ATP powers the enzymes Na^+--K^+ ATPase and Ca^{++}--Mg^{++} ATPase located within the cell wall to pump potassium into cells as it pumps sodium out.

This pumping creates a negative electrical charge needed on the cell wall. When oxidized or glycosylated, Na^+--K^+ ATPase can't do its job as well. With less activity in these mineral-transporting enzymes, cells have trouble bringing certain amino acids and minerals inside, where they can be used to build the enzymes and structures needed for good health. Poorly charged cells result, causing retention of sodium and weakening of the cell's ability to sort out what enters and what doesn't. This weakening of negative or anionic charge is one of the first changes found in people who later develop high blood pressure and kidney disease, but has been shown to be corrected by good control on an insulin pump.[140]

The aldose reductase (AR) pathway appears to be linked to loss of vitamin C. Both the intake of myoinositol and the AR inhibitor, Tolrestat, correct the low vitamin C levels seen in diabetes.[141] And a vitamin C supplement has been shown to lower cell sorbitol levels by as much as 50%.[142] A low magnesium level inside cells, frequently found in diabetes, also causes a loss of myoinositol. Magnesium is lost from cells in direct proportion to the blood sugar level. The higher the blood sugar, the lower the cell levels of magnesium, myoinositol, NAD+ and ATP. Hundreds of enzymes in the cell depend on having these to do their work. The drop in cell levels of these critical elements in a high blood sugar environment makes it hard for cells to thrive.

Vitamin C is needed to form normal protein structures in the body. Zinc, a mineral cofactor required by enzymes that make protein structures, is also lost from the body in increasing amounts as the blood sugar rises. The low concentrations of some amino acids, along with excess losses of magnesium, vitamin C and zinc create defective enzymes, cell membranes and DNA. Structures like blood vessels are affected since they are formed from these energy and structural elements, which are not as available in an environment of high blood sugars.

Myoinositol, ATP and NAD+ levels can be increased with drugs called aldose reductase (AR) and sorbitol dehydrogenase (SDH) inhibitors. Work is ongoing with a variety of these drugs to see if they will protect against nerve, kidney and eye damage found in diabetes, while not creating problems themselves. Although less powerful than AR and SDH inhibitors, the successes seen with myoinositol, bioflavanoids, and vitamin C offer some hope that effective methods to reduce damage caused by an overactive AR pathway will be found.

HOMOCYSTEINE

Homocysteine came into the limelight several years ago when researchers found that blood levels of this precursor to two amino acids were high in certain families who had a genetic risk for early heart attacks. First heart attacks usually occur in members of these families between the ages of 10 and 45 years. Some of these heart attack-prone families were discovered to have an enzyme deficiency that created high blood levels of homocysteine.[143]

This incidental finding became more intriguing when other researchers discovered that homocysteine directly damages blood vessels and is strongly associated with heart attacks, strokes and peripheral vascular disease.[144, 145] Homocysteine attaches to LDL and modifes it in a way that makes it more likely to cause heart disease.[146] In one study, homocysteine concentrations were found to be 4 times as high in the LDL of men who had high cholesterol levels compared to those who did not.[147] In another study of nearly 15,000 physicians, those who were in the top 5% for blood levels of homocysteine were **three and a half times** as likely to have a heart attack.[148]

Having a high homocysteine level due to an enzyme deficiency is rare, but blood levels of this compound also rise when B vitamin levels are low. Unfortunately, vitamin B deficiencies become more common as we age.[149] One study found one or more B vitamin deficiencies in 63% of healthy Europeans over the age of 65, and in 83% of the elderly who were hospitalized for any reason.[150] Excess urination caused by high blood sugars seems to be an additional risk factor for loss of these water-soluble vitamins. Homocysteine is found at high levels in most people with diabetes who have kidney disease,[151] and in 20% to 40% of the general population with heart disease.[152,153]

A buidup of homocysteine comes at the cost of lowered cysteine levels, which has important antioxidant properties. Cysteine levels were raised 50% in a study of 20 to 30 year old women given a vitamin B-6 supplement.[154] High levels of homocysteine also lower copper levels. Activity of superoxide dismutase as an antioxidant depends on copper[155] and its antioxidant activity may also help slow aging.[98] Luckily for most people, blood levels of homocysteine are easily lowered with a simple vitamin B complex. Fish oil has also been shown to decrease homocysteine levels.[156]

ESSENTIAL FATTY ACIDS AND OTHER FATS

Fat and sugar metabolism are tightly linked in the body's orchestration of energy flow. When blood sugars are high, problems in fatty acid metabolism begin to occur. Fats provide energy to cells, and at times excess body weight. Some fats, called essential fatty acids (EFAs), are building blocks for complex molecules that we need for health and are found largely in fish, seeds and plants. The human body requires these complex polyunsaturated fatty acids for the integrity of cell membranes and for the creation of hormone-like substances called prostaglandins and cytokines.

The excess glycosylation and oxidation found with high blood sugars damage enzymes needed to make EFAs, like delta-6-desaturase and delta-5-desaturase.[157] When these enzymes are inactivated, the body is less able to form EFAs, and their important byproducts. EFAs, prostaglandins and cytokines are needed to dilate and constrict blood vessels, reduce inflammation, and provide electrical insulation to nerve fibers that send messages through the body.

These Complex fatty acids also give a fluid motion to cell membranes. This motion is critical for enzymes to work and red blood cells to flex their way through the very tiny blood vessels that nourish nerves. A problem seen in diabetes is the absence of EFAs in cell membranes. And when EFAs are present, they are specifically targeted by the excess oxidation found in diabetes. The oxidation of EFAs makes cells stiffer, inactivates enzymes and causes blood vessels to harden. The abscence of EFAs together with the excess oxidative damage to them appears to cause nerve damage.[158] Finnish researchers have shown that improved blood sugar control on an insulin pump will correct these cell membrane deficits of EFAs.[159]

Cells have an outer wall or membrane that separates their interior from the exterior world around them. These cell membranes are composed mostly of fats in the form of phospholipids and triglycerides, together with some proteins and enzymes. Similar membranes on the interior of the cell separate important manufacturing sites, called the mitochondria and the endoplastic reticulum, from the rest of the cell. These membranes contain enzymes that perform functions vital to life, and for this reason membrane structure is critical to the activity of the enzymes that reside within them.

Some examples from among the hundreds of these enzymes in the cell membrane are sodium-potassium ATPase or Na^+--K^+ATPase, and calcium-magnesium ATPase or Ca^{++}--Mg^{++}ATPase, both mentioned earlier. The pumping action of these enzymes keeps **95% of the potassium and 90% of the magnesium inside the cell while similar amounts of sodium and calcium are kept on the outside**. This allows the cell to maintain a negative charge. Activities of both Na^+--K^+ ATPase and Ca^{++}ATPase have been shown to be lowered by oxidation (free radical damage).[160] **Lower activity** of Na^+--K^+ATPase has been noted years before people develop a number of diseases, like high blood pressure, elevated triglycerides, Type II diabetes, and diabetic kidney disease.

Obviously, healthy EFAs and other cell components are important to our health, just as the floor, roof and walls of a home are important. In early research studies, large doses of corn oil were used in an attempt to overcome the EFA defects found in diabetes. Some promising results occurred in treating eye disease,[161] but no one could tolerate a diet where most of the daily fat intake came from corn oil. As an understanding of the chemistry evolved, smaller doses of the fatty acid, gamma linolenic acid (GLA, an Omega-6 fatty acid), were shown to reverse nerve damage.[162] In a double-blind study that involved 113 people with diabetes for one year, treatment with GLA showed significant improvements in nerve function on 13 of 16 different nerve tests when compared to a placebo.[163]

Use of GLA is mildly controversial because it is also a precursor to the fatty acid, arachadonic acid, which is generally believed to be low in diabetes, but has been found to be higher than normal in some studies. Theoretically, excess arachadonic acid could contribute to arthritis and to abnormal clotting.

Cousins of GLA, the Omega-3 fatty acids found in seed and fish oils, look interesting as protective interventions. But the amounts used are important. Eating fish regularly or taking small doses of whole body fish oil appears to have favorable health effects. But larger doses (more than 5 capsules of fish oil per day, for instance), appear to cause insulin resistance and make insulin requirements rise. Seed oils do not appear to cause insulin resistance and can be obtained from raw pumpkin, flax, sesame, or sunflower seeds, or as flax seed oil. Because these highly unsaturated oils are more prone to oxidation, the intake of antioxidants to protect their structures is wise. Seeds have antioxidants built in, but fish have only a limited antioxidant content. An antioxidant supplement is particularly wise with regular fish intake.

Changes Related To The Heart And Blood Vessels

Besides the complications characteristic of diabetes, other health problems that occur among the general population tend to show up earlier and with increased frequency and severity in those with poorly controlled diabetes. Damage involving the heart and blood vessels are the most important of these accelerated diseases.

Complications involving the heart and blood vessels are linked to high blood sugar levels,[164] but less directly than eye, nerve, and kidney complications. Several interlinked mechanisms contribute to this vessel damage. When blood sugar levels are high, increases are seen in these risk factors for heart disease:

Lipid Changes

- LDL or "bad" cholesterol levels rise, increasing the risk of harmful deposits on blood vessel walls.[165]
- LDL is structurally modified by both excess oxidation and glycosylation. Only oxidized or glycated LDL will trigger the processes (uptake by macrophages and formation of foam cells) that create plaque.[166]
- HDL or "good" cholesterol is less efficient in doing its work to clean cholesterol deposits from blood vessel walls.
- Triglyceride and free fatty acid levels are increased, causing more oxidation and clotting.
- Lipid structures like triglycerides and LDL become smaller and heavier, causing them to deposit more easily within blood vessels. (Oils from fish help lighten them.)

Glycosylation and Oxidation

- Vitamins and minerals that work as antioxidants are lost or inactivated, leaving substances like LDL more prone to oxidation.
- Glycosylation of proteins within the blood vessel wall causes loss of elasticity and encourages cholesterol deposits.

Increased Clotting

- Blood thickens, making it harder for the heart to pump.
- Platelets and red blood cells clot easily, increasing the plugging of blood vessels.
- Levels of thromboxane, fibrinogen, and prostaglandins that cause clotting are higher.
- The outer surface of red cells becomes harder, creating more damage to the blood vessels through which they pass, causing additional closure of blood vessels.

Other

- Low levels of cell magnesium and high levels of oxidized fat increase risk for arrythmias.
- Growth hormone levels are increased, contributing to a rise in the number of cells involved in plaque formation.
- Levels of L-carnitine, a transporter for the free fatty acids on which the heart runs are lower. This lowers ATP levels and the activity of ATP-dependent enzymes, which may weaken the heart and other muscles.
- Higher histamine levels cause excessive leakage through blood vessels.

136

Signs that risks for heart disease and death can be lowered are showing promise in studies of the general population. The same preventive methods used in these studies are likely to help those who have diabetes, as the underlying causes appear to be identical, but simply increased in an environment of high blood sugars.

Two promising interventions involve the use of aspirin and of antioxidants. Studies of low-dose aspirin show a 17% to 44% reduction in the risk of a heart attack and a smaller (generally about 10%) reduction in the overall death rate due to its blood thinning properties.[167] Because of these benefits and no evidence of harmful effects from low dose aspirin, the Early Treatment of Diabetic Retinopathy Study Group recommended that aspirin be used by people with diabetes at risk for heart disease. (No particular benefit or harm was shown in the use of aspirin to treat eye disease in this large study, but the heart and lifespan benefits prompted this recommendation.)

The American Heart Association's Board of Directors does caution that on the "available data, the clinical decision to use aspirin in primary prevention should be made on an individual basis by a physician or other health care provider."[168] If you have any history of bleeding, stomach problems, stroke, asthma, or are using another blood thinner like coumadin or heparin, be sure to discuss aspirin use with your physician.

The actions of low dose aspirin and of antioxidants appear to be **complementary**. No large studies have tested both therapies, but their combined use may reduce the risk of heart attacks more than each used alone. Research is ongoing in this area and constantly being updated.

Successful strategies to prevent and reverse diabetes complications will only come from the use of multiple interventions, with each targeted at one or more of the different mechanisms through which damage occurs. There are too many mechanisms to cover in this chapter and only a few of the many mechanisms involved in diabetes complications have been discussed. But, as you can tell from the representative studies discussed here, researchers are slowly uncomplicating complications.

"When we talk to God, we're praying.
When God talks to us, we're schizophrenic."

Lily Tomlin

FINAL THOUGHTS

21

Controlling blood sugars is always individualized to a person's needs. The process involves learning more about who you are. In adding an insulin pump to your life, expect to encounter periods where you will meet new challenges. There is no way for you to master blood sugar control and pumping without learning from a few mistakes.

With any challenging situation like blood sugar control, problems with fine tuning are likely to occur. It helps to have the assistance of a knowledgeable support team. Pumps, like other advanced technology, work best when guided by a full array of professionals.

You are responsible for collecting and recording the information related to your blood sugars. But health professionals' trained eyes will spot important information and patterns in your charts that you may miss. Their experience allows them to quickly help you deal with the questions and problems that arise. How quickly you succeed on an insulin pump depends to a large extent on how well you use the knowledge and support of your physician/health care team.

Another helpful aid, if available in your community, is a support group. Support groups are made up of people who have diabetes, their relatives, friends and local health professionals. They provide an opportunity for everyone to catch up on the latest news in diabetes, and to help one another with advice and information. Support groups often help their members accept diabetes and deal with it more effectively. Other members understand the rewards and difficulties of having diabetes better than people outside the group who haven't shared your experiences.

If you have a support group available, join it for the friendship and information it provides. If none exists, consider forming one. You need no agenda, just the desire to know and share your experience with other people with diabetes.

We hope the information in this book helps you in using your pump. We learned a great deal in writing it. We tried to keep you, our reader, in mind as we wrote, hoping that we were providing this information in words and ways that would be the clearest for you to read and understand.

We give our wholehearted support for your efforts as you use your pump to improve your blood sugars and health. You've already come far, simply by engaging in this process. Our best to you on your adventure.

*"If your capacity to acquire has outstripped your capacity to enjoy,
you are on your way to the scrap-heap."*

Glen Buck

REFERENCES

[1] D. Fedele et. al.: Influence of continuous insulin infusion (CSII) treatment on diabetic somatic and autonomic neuropathy. *J. Endocrinol. Invest.* 7: 623-628, 1984.

[2] A.J. Boulton, J. Drury, B. Clarke, and J.D. Ward: Continuous subcutaneous insulin infusion in the management of painful diabetic neuropathy. *Diabetes Care* 5: 386-390, 1982.

[3] G. Viberti: Correction of exercise-induced microalbuminuria in insulin-dependent diabetics after 3 weeks of subcutaneous insulin infusion. *Diabetes* 30: 818-823, 1981.

[4] T. Olsen et. al.: Diabetic retinopathy after 3 years' treatment with continuous subcutaneous insulin infusion. *Acta Ophthalmol.* (Copenh) 65: 185-189, 1987.

[5] H.L. Eichner et. al.: Reduction of severe hypoglycemic events in Type I (insulin dependent) diabetic patients using continuous subcutaneous insulin infusion. *Diabetes Research* 8: 189-193, 1988.

[6] E. Chantelau, M. Spraul, I. Muhlhauser, et. al.: Long-term safety, efficacy and side-effects of continuous subcutaneous insulin infusion treatment for Type I (insulin-dependent) diabetes mellitus: a one center experience. *Diabetologia* 32: 421-426, 1989.

[7] H. Beck-Nielsen, B. Richelsen, C. Hasling, et. al.: Improved in vivo insulin effect during continuous subcutaneous insulin infusion in patients with IDDM. *Diabetes* 33: 832-837, 1984.

[8] A.O. Marcus: Patient selection for insulin pump therapy. *Practical Diabetology* (November, 1992) 12-18.

[9] C. Binder et al.: Insulin pharmacokinetics. *Diabetes Care* 7: 188-199, 1984.

[10] T. Lauritzen et al.: Pharmacokinetics of continuous subcutaneous insulin infusion. *Diabetologia* 24: 326-329, 1983.

[11] I. Lager et. al.: Reversal of insulin resistance in Type I diabetes after treatment with continuous subcutaneous insulin infusion. *BMJ* 287: 1661-1663, 1983.

[12] K. Dahl-Jorgensen et al.: Effect of near normoglycemia for two years on progression of early diabetic retinopathy, nephropathy, and neuropathy: the Oslo study. *BMJ* 293: 1195-1201, 1986.

[13] R.S. Mecklenburg et al.: Acute complications associated with insulin infusion pump therapy. *JAMA* 252: 3265-3269, 1984.

[14] J.J. Bending et al.: Complications of insulin infusion pump therapy. *JAMA* 253: 2644, 1985.

[15] The Diabetes Control and Complications Trial Research Group: The effect of intensive treatment of diabetes on the development and progression of long-term complications in insulin-dependent diabetes mellitus. *N Engl J Med* 329: 977-986, 1993.

[16] I.B. Hirsch, R. Farkas-Hirsch and P.D. Cryer: Continuous subcutaneous insulin infusion for the treatment of diabetic patients with hypoglycemic unawareness. *Diabetes Nutr. Metab.* 4: 1-3, 1991.

[17] R. Farkas-Hirsch and I.B. Hirsch: Continuous subcutaneous insulin infusion (CSII): A review of the past and its implementation for the future. Accepted for publication in March/April, 1994 issue of *Diabetes Spectrum*.

[18] C.G. Fanelli, L. Epifano, A.M. Rambotti, S. Pampanelli, A. DiVincenzo, F. Modarelli et. al.: Meticulous prevention of hypoglycemia normalizes the glycemic thresholds and magnitude of most of neuroendocrine responses to, symptoms of, and cognitive function during hypoglycemia in intensively treated patients with short-term IDDM. *Diabetes* 42: 1683-1689, 1993.

[19] L.C. Groop et al.: Risk factors and markers associated with proliferative retinopathy in patients with insulin-dependent diabetes. *Diabetes* 35: 1397-1403, 1986.

[20] R.L. Engerman and T.S. Kern: Hyperglycemia as a cause of diabetic retinopathy. *Metabolism* 35 (suppl. 1) 4: 20-23, 1986.

[21] T.R. Friberg, J. Rosenstock, G. Sanborn, A. Vaghefi and P. Raskin: The effect of long-term near normal glycemic control on mild diabetic retinopathy. *Ophthalmology* 92: 1051-1058, 1985.

[22] H. Beck-Nielsen, B. Richelsen, C.E. Mogensen, T. Olsen, N. Ehlers, C.B. Nielsen and P. Charles: Effect of insulin pump treatment for one year on renal and retinal morphology in patients with IDDM. *Diabetes Care* 8: 585-589, 1985.

[23] D.J. Ballard et al.: Epidemiology of persistent proteinuria in Type II Diabetes Mellitus. *Diabetes* 37: 405-412, 1988.

[24] H.P. Chase et al.: Glucose control and the renal and retinal complications of insulin-dependent diabetes. *JAMA* 261: 1155-1160, 1989.

[25] V. Frighi et al.: Early signs of neuropathy and microangiopathy in young Type I diabetic patients: correlation with long-term control. (Abstract) *Diabetologia* 30: 521A, 1987.

[26] J. Jakobsen et al.: Autonomic and somatosensory nerve fuction after 2 years of continuous subcutaneous insulin infusion in Type I diabetes. *Diabetes* 37: 452-455, 1988.

[27] A. Schiffrin and M. Belmonte: Multiple daily self-glucose monitoring: its essential role in long-term glucose control in insulin-dependent diabetic patients treated with pump and multiple subcutaneous injections. *Diabetes Care* 5: 479-484, 1982.

[28] H.U. Janka, J.H. Warram, L.I. Rand and A.S.Krolewski: Risk factors for progression of background retinopathy in long-standing IDDM. *Diabetes* 38: 460-464, 1989.

139

[29] L.C. Groop et al.: Risk factors and markers associated with proliferative retinopathy in patients with insulin-dependent diabetes. *Diabetes* 35: 1397-1403, 1986.

[30] E. Chantelau, H Weiss, U. Weber, G.E. Sonnenberg, and M. Berger: Four-year followup of retinal status and glycosylated hemoglobin in patients with insulin-dependent diabetes mellitus. *Diabete & Metabolisme* 14: 259-263, 1988.

[31] J. Pirart: Diabetes Mellitus and its degenerative complications: A prospective study of 4,400 patients observed between 1947 and 1973. *Diabetes Care* 1: 168-188, 1978.

[32] S.D. Prato and A. Tiengo: Pancreatic diabetes. *Diabetes Reviews* 1: 260-285, 1993.

[33] K. Dahl-Jorgensen et al.: Reduction of urinary albumin excretion after 4 years of continuous insulin infusion in insulin-dependent diabetes mellitus. *NEJM* 316: 1376-1383, 1987.

[34] W. Troni et al.: Peripheral nerve function and metabolic control in diabetes mellitus. *Ann. Neurol.* 16: 178-183, 1984.

[35] H.H. Parving et. al.: Prevalence of microalbuminuria, arterial hypertension, retinopathy and neuropathy in patients with insulin-dependent diabetes. *BMJ* 296: 156-160, 1988.

[36] D.J. Ballard et. al.: Epidemiology of persistent proteinuria in Type II diabetes mellitus: Population-based study in Rochester, Minnesota. *Diabetes* 37: 405-412, 1988.

[37] D.G. Warnock and F.C. Rector: Treatment of Renal Disease in the Diabetic. Upjohn Medical Education Series 11: 6, 1987.

[38] G.C. Viberti et. al.: Effect of control of blood glucose on urinary excretion of albumin and B2-microglobulin in insulin-dependent diabetes. *NEJM* 300: 638-641, 1979.

[39] M. Brownlee: Glycation products and the pathogenesis of diabetic complications. *Diabetes Care* 15: 1835-1843, 1992.

[40] J. Sattler and W. Lorenz: Intestinal diamine oxidases and enteral-induced histaminosis: studies on three prognostic variables in an epidemiological model. *J. Neural. Transm. Suppl.* 32: 291-314, 1990.

[41] I. Lager et. al.: Reversal of insulin resistance in Type I diabetes after treatment with continuous subcutaneous insulin infusion. *BMJ* 287: 1661-1663, 1983.

[42] H. Beck-Nielsen et. al.: Improved in vivo insulin effect during continuous subcutaneous insulin infusion in patients with IDDM. *Diabetes* 33: 832-837, 1984.

[43] E. Van Ballegooie, J.M. Hooymans, Z. Timmerman, et. al.: Rapid deterioration of diabetic retinopathy during treatment with continuous subcutaneous insulin infusion. *Diabetes Care* 7:236-242, 1984.

[44] D. Dahl-Jorgensen, O. Brinchmann-Hansen, K.F. Hansen, et. al.: Transient deterioration of retinopathy when multiple insulin injection therapy and CSII is started in IDDM patients. *Diabetes* 33(1): 4A, 1984.

[45] R.S. Mecklenburg and T.S. Guinn: Complications of insulin pump therapy: The effect of insulin preparation. *Diabetes Care* 8: 367-370, 1985.

[46] S.G. Melberg, S. Havelund, J. Villumsen, and J. Brange: Insulin compatibility with polymer materials used in external pump infusion systems. *Diabetic Medicine* 5: 243-247, 1988.

[47] V.A. Koivisto and P. Felig: Alterations in insulin absorption and in blood glucose control associated with varying insulin injection sites in diabetic patients. *Ann. Intern. Med.* 92: 59-61, 1980.

[48] J.P. Bantle et al.: Rotation of the anatomic regions used for insulin injections and day-to-day variability of plasma glucose in Type I diabetic subjects. *JAMA* 263: 1802-1806, 1990.

[49] V.A. Koivisto and P. Felig: Effect of leg exercise on insulin absorption in diabetic patients. *NEJM* 298: 79-83, 1978.

[50] A. Pietri and P. Raskin: Cutaneous complications of chronic continuous subcutaneous insulin infusion therapy. *Diabetes Care* 4: 624-627, 1981.

[51] M.H. Tanner et. al.: Toxic shock syndrome from staphylococcus areus infection at insulin pump infusion sites. *JAMA* 259: 394-395, 1988.

[52] A. Schiffrin and M. Belmonte: Multiple daily self-glucose monitoring: its essential role in long-term glucose control in insulin-dependent patients treated with pump and multiple subcutaneous injections. *Diabetes Care* 5: 479-484, 1982.

[53] J.S. Christiansen et. al.: Clinical outcome of using insulin at 40 IU/ml and 100 IU/ml in pump treatment. Results of a controlled multi-center trial. *Acta Med. Scan.* 221: 385-393, 1987.

[54] J. Beyer et. al.: Assessment of insulin needs in insulin-dependent diabetics and healthy volunteers under fasting conditions. *Horm. Metab. Res. Suppl.* 24: 71-77, 1990.

[55] W. Bruns et. al.: Nocturnal continuous subcutaneous insulin infusion: a therapeutic possibility in labile Type I diabetes under exceptional conditions. *Z. Gesamte Inn. Med.* 45: 154-158, 1990.

[56] K. Haakens et. al.: Early morning glycaemia and the metabolic consequences of delaying breakfast/morning insulin. A comparison of continuous subcutaneous insulin infusion and multiple injection therapy with human isophane or human Ultralente at bedtime. *Scand. J. Clin. Lab. Invest.* 49: 653-659, 1989.

[57] G. Perriello, P. De Feo, E. Torlone, et. al.: The Dawn Phenomenon in Type I (insulin-dependent) diabetes mellitus; magnitude, frequency, variability, and dependency on glucose counterregulation and insulin sensitivity. *Diabetologia* 42: 21-28, 1991.

[58] P. Hildebrandt, K. Birch, B.M. Jensen, and C. Kuhl: Subcutaneous insulin infusion: Change in basal infusion rate has no immediate effect on insulin absorption rate. *Diabetes Care* 9: 561-564, 1986.

[59] H. Beck-Nielsen et. al.: Improved in vivo insulin effect during continuous subcutaneous insulin infusion in patients with IDDM. *Diabetes* 33: 832-837, 1984.

[60] G. Perriello, P. De Feo, E. Torlone, et. al.: Nocturnal spikes of growth hormone secretion cause the dawn phenomenon in Type I (insulin-dependent) diabetes mellitus by decreasing hepatic (and extra-hepatic) sensitivity to insulin in the absence of insulin waning. *Diabetologia* 33(1): 52-59, 1990.

[61] J.M. Stephenson et al.: Dawn Phenomenon and Somogyi Effect in IDDM. *Diabetes Care* 12: 245-251, 1989.

[62] B. Zinman: The physiologic replacement of insulin. *NEJM* 321: 363-370, 1989.

[63] N. Perrotti, D. Santoro, S. Genovese et al.: Effect of digestible carbohydrates on glucose control in insulin-dependent diabetic patients. *Diabetes Care* 7: 354-359, 1984.

[64] G. Boden and F. Jadali: Effects of lipid on basal carbohydrate metabolism in normal men. *Diabetes* 40: 686-692, 1991.

[65] D.M. Mott, S. Lilloija, and C. Bogardus: Overnutrition induced decrease in insulin action for glucose storage: in vivo and in vitro in man. *Metabolism* 35: 160-165, 1986.

[66] E. Ferrannini, E.J. Barrett, S. Bevilacqua, R.A. DeFronzo: Effect of fatty acids on glucose production and utilization in man. *J. Clin. Invest.* 1983; 72: 1737-1747.

[67] G.M. Reaven: Banting Lecture 1988: Role of insulin resistance in human disease. *Diabetes* 37: 1595-1607, 1988.

[68] P. Halfon, J. Belkhadir and G. Slama: Correlation between amount of carbohydrate in mixed meals and insulin delivery by artificial pancreas in seven IDDM subjects. *Diabetes Care* 12: 427-429, 1989.

[69] F.Q. Nuttall, A.D. Mooradian, M.C. Gannon et al.: Effect of protein ingestion on the glucose and insulin response to a standardized oral glucose load. *Diabetes Care* 7: 465-470, 1984.

[70] D. Cox, L. Gonder-Frederick, W. Polonsky, D. Schlundt, B. Kovatchev and W. Clark: Recent hypoglycemia influences the probability of subsequent hypoglycemia in Type I patients. Abstract 399, ADA Conference 1993.

[71] A. Avogaro, P. Beltramello, L. Gnudi, A. Maran, A. Valerio, M. Miola, N. Marin, C. Crepaldi, L. Confortin, F. Costa, I. MacDonald and A. Tiengo: Alcohol intake impairs glucose counterregulation during acute insulin-induced hypoglycemia in IDDM patients. *Diabetes* 42: 1626-1634, 1993.

[72] T. Veneman, A. Mitrakou, M. Mokan, P. Cryer and J. Gerich: Induction of hypoglycemia unawareness by asymptomatic nocturnal hypoglycemia. *Diabetes* 42: 1233-1237, 1993.

[73] C.G. Fanelli, L. Epifano, A.M. Rambotti, S. Pampanelli, A. Di Vincenzo, F. Modarelli, M. Lepore, B Annibale, M. Ciofetta, P. Bottini, F. Porcellati, L. Scionti, F. Santeusanio, P. Brunetti and G.B. Bolli: Meticulous prevention of hypoglycemia normalizes the glycemic thresholds and magnitude of most of neuroendocrine responses to, symptoms of, and cognitive function during hypoglycemia in intensively treated patients with short-term IDDM. *Diabetes* 42: 1683-1688, 1993.

[74] E.S. Horton: Role and management of exercise in Diabetes Mellitus. *Diabetes Care* 11: 201-211, 1988.

[75] K. E. Powell et al.: Physical activity and chronic disease. *Am J. Clin. Nutr.* 49: 999-1006, 1989.

[76] K.J. Cruickshanks, R.Klein, S.E. Moss, and B.E.K. Klein: Physical activity and proliferative retinopathy in people diagnosed with diabetes before age 30 yr. *Diabetes Care* 15: 1267-1272, 1992.

[77] J. Wahren: Glucose turnover during exercise in healthy man and in patients with Diabetes Mellitus. *Diabetes* 28(1): 82-88, 1979.

[78] P. Felig and J. Wahren: Role of insulin and glucagon in the regulation of hepatic glucose production during exercise. *Diabetes* 28(1): 71-75, 1979.

[79] P. Micossi et. al.: Free-insulin profiles after intraperitoneal, intramuscular, and subcutaneous insulin administration. *Diabetes Care* 9: 575-578, 1986.

[80] J.A. Ahern, P.M. Gatcomb, N.A. Held, W.A. Petit, W.V. Tamborlane: Exaggerated hyperglycemia after pizza meal in well-controlled diabetes. *Diabetes Care* 16: 578-580, 1993.

[81] J. Stamler, O. Vaccaro, J.D. Neaton and D. Wentworth: Diabetes, other risk factors, and 12-year cardiovascular mortality for men screened in the Multiple Risk Factor Intervention Trial. *Diabetes Care* 16: 434-444, 1993.

[82] A. Cerami, H. Vlassara and M. Brownlee: Glucose and aging. *Scientific American* 256 (5): 90-96, May 1987.

[83] J.R. Williamson, K. Chang, M. Frangos, K.S. Hasan, Y. Ido, T. Kawamura, J.R. Nyengaard, M. Van Den Enden, C. Kilo, and R. G. Tilton: Hyperglycemic pseudohypoxia and diabetic complications. *Diabetes* 42: 801-813, 1993.

[84] R.L. Engerman and T.S. Kern: Aldose reductase inhibition fails to prevent retinopathy in diabetic and galactosemic dogs. *Diabetes* 42: 820-825, 1993.

[85] R.N. Frank: Perspectives in diabetes: the aldose reductase controversy. *Diabetes* 43: 169-172, 1994.

[86] A. Cerami et. al.: Role of advanced glycosylation products in complications of diabetes. *Diabetes Care* 11 (Supplement 1): 73-79, 1988.

[87] H. Vlassara, M. Brownlee and A. Cerami: Recognition and uptake of human peripheral nerve myelin by macrophages. *Diabetes* 34: 553-557, 1985.

88 V.M. Monnier, V. Vishwanath, R.E. Frank, C. Elmets, P. Dauchot and R.R. Kohn: Relations between complications to Type I diabetes mellitus and collagen-linked flourescence. *N. Engl. J. Med.* 314: 403-408, 1986.

89 A.L. Rosenbloom, D. Schatz and J.H. Silverstein: Joint disease in diabetes mellitus. *Practical Diabetology* 11:4-8, 1992.

90 A. Ceriello, D. Giugliano, A. Quatraro and P. Dello Russo: Metabolic control may influence the increased superoxide generation in diabetic serum. *Diab. Med.* 8: 540-542, 1991.

91 A.H. Schapira and J.M. Cooper: Mitochondrial function in neurodegeneration and aging. *Mutat. Res.* 275: 133-143, 1992.

92 K.D. Gerbitz: Does the mitochondrial DNA play a role in the pathogenesis of diabetes? *Diabetologia* 35: 1181-1186, 1992.

93 R. Bucala, Z. Makita, T Koschinsky, H. Fuh and H. Vlassara: Advanced glycosylation of the apoprotein and lipid components of LDL reflects the number and severity of diabetic complications. *Diabetes* 42: 119A, 1993.

94 M. Hogan, A. Cerami and R. Bucala: Advanced glycosylation endproducts block the antiproliferative effect of nitric oxide: Role in the vascular and renal complications of diabetes mellitus. *J. Clin. Invest.* 90: 1110-1115, 1992.

95 T. Deckert, A. Kofoed-Enevoldsan, K. Norgaard, K. Borch-Johnsen, B. Feldt-Rasmussen and T. Jensen: Microalbuminuria. *Diabetes Care* 15: 1181-1191, 1992.

96 M. Sensi, M.G. De Rossi, F.S. Celi, A. Cristina, C. Rosati, D. Perrett, D. Andreani and U. Di Mario: D-lysine reduces non-enzymatic glycation of proteins in experimental diabetes mellitus in rats. *Diabetologia* 36: 797-801, 1993.

97 M. Fu, K.J. Knecht, S.R. thorpe and J.W. Baynes: Role of oxygen in cross-linking and chemical modification of collagen by glucose. *Diabetes* 41 (suppl. 2): 42-48, 1992.

98 R.L. Rusting: Why do we age? *Scientific American* 12: 130-141, December 1992.

99 B.K. Siesjo: Cell damage in the brain: a speculative synthesis. *J. Cereb. Blood Flow Metabol.* 1: 155-185, 1981.

100 D. Harman, S. Hendricks, D.E. Eddy, and J. Seibold: Free radical theory of aging: effect of dietary fat on central nervous system function. *J. Amer. Geriatrics Soc.* July vol. 24, July, 1976.

101 G.V. Mann: *Perspect. Biol. Med.* 17: 210-217, 1974.

102 Y. Sato, N Hotta, N. Sakamoto, S. Matsuoka, N. Ohishi and K. Yage: Lipid peroxide levels in plasma of diabetic patients. *Biochem. Med.* 21: 104-107, 1979.

103 I. Nishigaki, M. Hagihara, H. Tsunekawa, M. Maseki and K. Yagi: Lipid peroxide levels of serum lipoprotein fractions of diabetic patients. *Biochem. Med.* 25: 373-378, 1981.

104 E.K. Illing, C.H. Gray and R.D. Lawrence: Blood glutathione and non-glucose substances in diabetes. *Biochem. J.* 48: 637-640, 1951.

105 C.W. Karpen, S. Cataland, T.M. O'Dorisio and R.V. Panganamala: Interrelation of platelet vitamin E and thromboxane synthesis in Type I diabetes mellitus. *Diabetes* 33: 239-243, 1984.

106 J.J. Strain: Disturbances of micronutrient and antioxidant status in diabetes. *Proceed. Nutr. Soc.* 50: 591-604, 1991.

107 E. Havivi, H.B. On and A. Reshef: Vitamins and trace metals status in NIDDM. *Inter. J. Vit. Nutr. Res.* 61: 328-333, 1991.

108 J.J. Cunningham et al: Reduced mononuclear leukocyte ascorbic acid content in adults with insulin-dependent diabetes mellitus consuming adequate dietary vitamin C. *Metabolism* 40: 146-149, 1991.

109 R.A. Riemersma, D.A. Wood, C.C.A. Macintyre, R.A. Elton, K.F. Gey and M.F. Oliver: *Lancet* 337: 1-5.

110 K.F. Gey: The antioxidant hypothesis of cardiovascular disease: epidemiology and mechanisms. *Biochem. Soc. Trans.* 18: 1041-1045, 1990

111 M.G.L. Hertog, E.M.J. Feskens, P.C.H. Hollman, M.B. Katan and D. Kromhout: Dietary antioxidant flavanoids and risk of coronary heart disease: the Zutphen Elderly Study. *Lancet* 342: 1007-1011, 1993.

112 M.J. Gaziano: Presentation at the American Heart Association 63rd Annual Scientific Session, 1990.

113 M.J. Stampfer, C.H. Hennekens, J.E. Manson, G.A. Colditz, B. Rosner and W.C. Willett: Vitamin E consumption and the risk of coronary disease in women. *N. Engl. J. Med.* 328: 1444-1449, 1993.

114 E.B. Rimm, M.J. Stampfer, A. Ascherio, E. Giovannucci, G.A. Colditz and W.C. Willett: Vitamin E consumption and the risk of coronary disease in men. *N. Engl. J. Med.* 328: 1450-1456, 1993.

115 J.E. Enstrom, L.E. Kanim and M.A. Klein: Vitamin C intake and mortality among a sample of the United States population. *Epidemiology* 3: 194-202, 1992.

116 R.H. Nagaraj, D.R. Sell, M. Prabhakaram, B.J. Ortwerth and V.M. Monnier: High correlation between pentosidine protein crosslinks and pigmentation implicates ascorbate in human lens senescence and cataractogenesis. *Proc. Nat. Acad. Sci. USA* 88: 10257-10261, 1991.

117 S.K. Jain and R. McVie: Effect of glycemic control on reduced glutathione levels in red blood cells of Type I diabetics. Abstract 662, American Diabetes Meeting 1992.

118 C.S. Johnston, C.G. Meyer and J.C. Srilakshmi: Vitamin C elevates red blood cell glutathione in healthy adults. *Am. J. Clin. Nutr.* 58: 103-105, 1993.

119 G. Paolisso, A. D'Amore, D. Giugliano, A. Ceriello, M. Varicchio and F. D'Onofrio: Pharmacologic doses of vitamin E improve insulin action in healthy subjects and noninsulin-dependent diabetic patients. *Am. J. Clin. Nutr.* 57: 650-656, 1993.

142

[120] G. Block: Vitamin C and reduced mortality. *Epidemiology* 3: 189-191, 1992.

[121] G. Block et al: Carcinogenesis. *Nutrition and Cancer* 18: 1-29, July-August, 1992.

[122] C. Mullarkey, D. Edelstein and M. Brownlee: Free radical generation by early glycation products: A mechanism for accelerated atherogenesis in diabetes. *Biochem. Biophy. Res. Comm.* 173: 932-939, 1990.

[123] S.J. Davie, B.J. Gould and J.S. Yudkin: Effect of vitamin C on glycosylation of proteins. *Diabetes* 41: 167-173, 1992.

[124] G. Paolisso, A. D'Amore, D. Galzerano, V. Balbi, D. Giugliano, M. Varicchio and F. D'Onofrio: Daily vitamin E supplements improve metabolic control but not insulin secretion in elderly Type II diabetic patients. *Diabetes Care* 16: 1433-1437, 1993.

[125] A. Ceriello, D. Giugliano, A. Quatraro, C. Donzella, G. Dipalo and P.J. Lefebvre: Vitamin E reduction of protein glycosylation in diabetics: new prospect for prevention of diabetic complications *Diab. Care* 14: 68-72, 1991.

[126] J.V. Hunt, C.C.T. Smith and S.P. Wolff: Autooxidative glycosylation and possible involvement of peroxides and free radicals in LDL modification by glucose. *Diabetes* 39: 1420-1424, 1990.

[127] S.K. Jain and R. Mc Vie: Effect of glycemic control on reduced glutathione levels in red blood cells of Type I diabetes. Abstract 662, American Diabetes Association Meeting, San Antonio, Tx. 1992.

[128] A.J.Sinclair, A.J. Girling, L. Gray, J. Lunec and A.H. Barnett: Disturbed handling of ascorbic acid in diabetic patients with and without microangiopathy during high dose ascorbate supplementation. *Diabetologia* 34: 171-175, 1991.

[129] A.J. Sinclair, A.J. Girling, L. Gray and C. LeGuen: An investigation of the relationship between free radical activity and vitamin C metabolism in elderly diabetic subjects with retinopathy. *Gerontology* 38: 268-274, 1992.

[130] J. Watanabe, F. Umeda, H. Wakasugi and H. Ibayashi: Effect of vitamin E on platelet aggregation in diabetes melitus. *Thromb. Haemostas.* 51: 313-316, 1984.

[131] C. Gisinger, J. Jeremy, P. Speiser, D. Mikhailidis, P. Dandona and G. Schernthaner: Effect of vitamin E supplementation on platelet thromboxane A2 production in Type I diabetic patients. *Diabetes* 37: 1260-1264, 1988.

[132] I. Ozden, G. Deniz, E. Tasali, A. Ulusarac, T. Altug and S. Buyukdevrim: The effect of vitamin E on glycosylated hemoglobin levels in diabetic rats: a preliminary report. *Diabetes Research* 12: 123-124, 1989.

[133] K. Arai, S. Iizuka, K. Oikawa and N. Taniguchi: *Biochim. Biophys. Acta.* 924: 292-296, 1987a.

[134] J.W. Baynes: Role of oxidative stress in development of complications in diabetes. *Diabetes* 40:405-412, 1991.

[135] K. Hiramatsu and S. Arimori: Increased superoxide production by mononuclear cells of patients with hypertriglyceridemia and diabetes. *Diabetes* 37: 832-837, 1988

[136] M. Kitahara, H.J. Eyre, R.E. Lynch et. al.: Metabolic activity of diabetic monocytes. *Diabetes* 29: 251-256, 1980.

[137] M. Doly, M.T. Droy-Lefaix and P. Braquet: Oxidative stress in the diabetic retina. *EXS* 62: 299-307, 1992.

[138] Editorial Board: Our vitamin prescription: the big four. *University of California at Berkeley Wellness Letter* 10(4): 1-5, 1994.

[139] W. Kahler, B. Kuklinski, C. Ruhlmann and C. Plotz: Diabetes mellitus: a free radical-associated disease. Results of adjuvant antioxidant supplementation. *Z. Gesamte Inn. Med.* 48: 223-232, 1993.

[140] H.J. Bangstad, A. Kofoed-Enevoldsen, K. Dahl-Jorgensen and K.F. Hanssen: Glomerular charge selectivity and the influence of improved blood glucose control in Type I (insulin-dependent) diabetic patients with microalbuminuria. *Diabetologia* 35: 1165-1169, 1992.

[141] D.K. Yue, S. McLennan, E. Fisher, S. Heffernan, C. Capogreco, G.R. Ross and J.R. Turtle: Ascorbic acid metabolism and polyol pathway in diabetes. *Diabetes* 38: 257-261, 1989.

[142] J.A. Vinson, M.E. Staretz, P. Bose, H.M. Kassm and B.S. Basalyga: In vitro and in vivo reduction of erythrocyte sorbitol by ascorbic acid. *Diabetes* 38: 1036-1041, 1989.

[143] J.B. Gibson, N. Carson, D.W. Neil: Pathological findings in homocystinuria. *J. Clin. Pathol.* 17: 427-437, 1964.

[144] K.S. McCully: Vascular pathology of homocysteinemia: implications for the pathogenisis of arteriosclerosis. *Am. J. Pathol.* 56: 111-128, 1969.

[145] K.S. McCully: Homocystinuria, arteriosclerosis, methylmalonic aciduria, and methyltransferase deficiency: a key case revisited. *Nutr. Rev.* 50: 7-12, 1992.

[146] A.J. Olszewski and K.S. McCully: Homocysteine metabolism and the oxidative modification of proteins and lipids. *Free Rad. Biol. Med.* 14: 683-693, 1993.

[147] A.J. Olszewski and K.S. McCully: Homocysteine content of lipoproteins in hypercholesterolemia. *Atherosclerosis* 88: 61-68, 1991.

[148] M.J. Stampfer, M.R. Malinow, W.C. Willet, L.M. Newcomer, B. Upson, D. Ullmann, P.V. Tishler and C.H. Hennekens: A prospective study of plasma homocysteine and risk of myocardial infarction in U.S. physicians. *JAMA* 268: 877-881, 1992.

[149] J.B. Ubbink, W.J.H. Vermaak, A. Van Der Merwe and P.J. Becker, D.A.: Vitamin B12, vitamin B6, and folate nutritional status in men with hyperhomocysteinemia. *Am. J. Clin. Nutr.* 57: 47-53, 1993.

[150] E. Joosten, A. van den Berg, R. Riezler, H.J. Naurath, J. Lindenbaum, S.P. Stabler and R.H. Allen: Metabolic evidence that deficiencies of vitamin B-12 (cobalamin), folate, and vitamin B-6 occur commonly in elderly people. *Am. J. Clin. Nutr.* 58: 468-476, 1993.

[151] B. Hultberg, E. Agardh, A. Andersson, L. Brattstrom et. al.: Increased levels of plasma homocysteine are associated with nephropathy, but not severe retinopathy in Type I diabetes mellitus. *Scand. J. Clin. Lab. Invest.* 51: 277-282. 1991.

[152] J.B. Ubbink, W.J.H. Vermaak, J.M. Bennett, P.J. Becker, D.A. Van Staden and S. Bissbort: The prevalence of homocysteinemia and hypercholesterolemia in angiographically defined coronary heart disease. *Klin. Wochenschr.* 69: 527-534, 1991.

[153] R. Clarke, L. Daly, K. Robinson, et. al.: Hyperhomocysteinemia: an independent risk factor for vascular disease. *N. Engl. J. Med.* 324: 1149-1155, 1991.

[154] S.A. Kang-Yoon and A. Kirksey: Relation of short-term pyridoxine-HCL supplementation to plasma vitamin B-6 vitamers and amino acid concentrations in young women. *Am. J. Clin. Nutr.* 55: 865-872, 1992.

[155] J.C.W. Brown and J.J. Strain: Effects of dietary homocysteine on copper status in rats. *J. Nutr.* 120: 1068-1074, 1990.

[156] A.J. Olszewski and K.S. McCully: Fish oil decreases serum homocysteine in hyperlipemic men. *Coron. Artery Dis.* 4: 53-60, 1993.

[157] J.P. Poisson: Comparative in vivo and in vitro study of the influence of experimental diabetes on rat liver linoleic acid 6- and 5-desaturation. *Enzyme* 34: 1-14, 1985.

[158] D.F. Horrobin: The effects of gamma-linolenic acid on breast pain and diabetic neuropathy: possible non-eicosanoid mechanisms. *Prostaglandins, Leukotrienes and Essential Fatty Acids* 48: 101-104, 1993.

[159] R.S. Tilvis, E. Helve and T.A. Miettinen: Improvment of diabetic control by continuous subcutaneous insulin infusion therapy changes fatty acid composition of serum lipids and erythrocytes in Type I (insulin-dependent) diabetes. *Diabetologia* 29: 690-694, 1986.

[160] M. Kaneko, P.K. Singal and N.S. Dhalla: Alterations in heart sarcolemmal Ca^{++}-ATPase and Ca^{++}-binding activities due to oxygen free radicals. *Basic Res. Cardiol.* 85: 45-54, 1990.

[161] A.J. Houtsmuller, K.J. Zahn and H.E. Henkes: Unsaturated fats and progression of diabetic retinopathy. *Doc. Ophthalmol.* 48: 363-371, 1979.

[162] G.A. Jamal and H. Carmichael: The effect of gamma-linolenic acid on human diabetic peripheral neuropathy: A double-blind placebo-controlled trial. *Diabetic Medicine* 7: 319-323, 1990.

[163] H. Keen, J. Payan, J. Allawi et al.: Treatment of diabetic neuropathy with gamma linolenic acid. *Diabetes Care* 16: 8-15, 1993.

[164] J.A. Colwell et al.: Pathogenesis of atherosclerosis in Diabetes Mellitus. *Diabetes Care* 4: 121-133 1981.

[165] F.L. Dunn et al.: Plasma lipid and lipoprotein levels with continuous subcutaneous insulin infusion in Type I Diabetes Mellitus. *Ann. Int. Med.* 95: 426-431, 1981.

[166] D. Steinberg, S. Parthasarathy, T.E. Carew, J.C. Khoo and J.L. Witztum: Beyond cholesterol. Modifications of low density lipoprotein that increase its atherogenicity. *New Engl. J. Med.* 320: 915-924, 1989.

[167] ETDRS Investigators: Aspirin effects on mortality and morbidity in patients with diabetes mellitus: Early Treatment Diabetic Retinopathy Study Report 14. *JAMA* 268: 1292-1300, 1992.

[168] V. Fuster, M.L. Dyken, P.S. Vokonas and C. Hennekens: AHA Medical/Scientific Statement: Aspirin as a therapeutic agent in cardiovascular disease. *Circulation* 87: 659-671, 1993.

CARBOHYDRATE COUNTING & FACTORS

APPENDIX A

HOW TO USE THIS GUIDE:

Few foods, other than table sugar and lollipops, are totally carbohydrate. So the Carbohydrate Factors for a variety of foods are provided on the following pages. These Factors give the amount of carbohydrate in 1 gram of that particular food. To find out how much carbohydrate you are eating in a particular food, you will need to do a simple calculation:

1. Weigh the food on a gram scale to get its total weight.
2. Then find that food and its Carbohydrate Factor in one of the Food Groups listed below.
3. On a calculator, multiply the food's weight in grams by its Carbohydrate Factor.
4. The answer is the number of grams of carbohydrate you are eating.

EXAMPLE:

Let's say you place a small apple on a gram scale and find that it weighs 100 grams. You then look up its Carbohydrate Factor and find that it is .13. You then simply multiply 100 grams by .13 to get the amount of carbohydrate you will be eating:

100 grams of apple X .13 = 13 grams of carbohydrate

ADDITIONAL INFORMATION:

These Carbohydrate Factors give the actual concentration of carbohydrate in foods. For instance, apples are 13% carbohydrate (most of their weight is water), while raisins are 77% carbohydrate by weight, and bagels contain 56% carbohydrate by weight. Both apple juice and regular sodas are 12% carbohydrate, although the carbohydrate in apple juice is higher in fructose, while a regular soda has more of its carbohydrate as sucrose or sugar.

Cranberry juice is even richer in carbohydrate at 16%, while grapefruit juice contains only 9% by weight. A 6-oz. glass of cranberry juice will therefore contain almost twice as much carbohydrate as an identical glass of grapefruit juice. Because it contains more carbohydrate, the glass of cranberry juice can raise the blood sugar nearly twice as far as the same amount of grapefruit juice. It will also require almost twice as much insulin to cover it.

Beverages

carbonated soda	.12	eggnog	.08	milk	.04
chocolate milk	.11	flavored instant coffee	.06	punch	.11

Alcoholic Beverages

beer: regular	.04	champagne	.01	wine: dry	.04
light	.02	liqueurs	.30	sweet	.12

Gin, rum, scotch, whiskey and vodka contain no carbohydrate. With 2 or more drinks, alcohol can lower the normal production of sugar by the liver. Because of the risk of a low blood sugar, no insulin is usually taken for alcoholic drinks. Discuss with your physician/health care team.

Breads & Grains

bagel	.56	french toast	.26	rice, cooked	.24
barley, uncooked	.77	lentils	.19	rolls	.60
biscuits	.45	macaroni: plain	.23	spaghetti: plain	.26
bread	.53	cheese	.20	with sauce	.15
bread crumbs	.74	muffins	.45	toast	.70
bread sticks	.75	pancakes & waffles:		tortillas: corn	.42
corn starch	.83	dry mix	.70	flour	.58
English muffin	.51	prepared	.44	wheat flour	.76

Dry Cold Cereals

All Bran	.78	Grapenuts	.83	Shredded Wheat	.81
Cheerios	.70	NutriGrain	.86	Special K	.76
Corn Chex	.89	Product 19	.84	Rice Krispies	.88
Corn Flakes	.84	Puffed Wheat	.77	Total	.79
Fruit and Fiber	.78	Raisin Bran	.75	Wheaties	.80
granola	.68	Quaker 100% Natural	.64		

Cooked Hot Cereals

corn grits	.11	oatmeal	.10	Wheatena	.12
Cream of Wheat	.14	Roman Meal	.14	Wheat Hearts	.12
Farina	.11				

Combination Dishes

beef stew	.06	coleslaw	.14	potato salad	.13
burrito	.24	fish & chips	.18	spaghetti & meat sauce	.15
chicken pie	.17	lasagna	.16	tossed salad	.05
chili with beans	.11	macaroni & cheese	.20	tuna casserole	.13
chili without beans	.06	pizza	.28		

Desserts and Sweets

apple butter	.46	cookies		ice milk	.23
banana bread	.47	animal	.80	jams	.70
brownie with nuts	.50	chocolate chip	.59	jellies	.70
cakes		fig bar	.71	pies	
angel food	.60	gingersnap	.80	apple	.37
coffee	.52	oatmeal & raisin	.72	blueberry	.34
fruit	.57	danish pastries	.46	cherry	.38
sponge	.55	doughnuts		lemon meringue	.38
candies		cake	.52	pecan	.23
caramel	.76	jelly filled	.46	pumpkin	.23
fudge with nuts	.69	fruit turnovers	.26	preserves	.70
hard	.96	honey	.76	sherbert	.32
jelly beans	.93	ice cream			
lollipops	1.00	plain	.21		
peanut brittle	.73	cone	.30		
chocolate syrup	.65	bar	.25		

Dressings, Sauces and Condiments

bacon bits	.19	olives	.04	pickle relish, sweet	.34
barbecue sauce	.13	pickles, sweet	.36	soy sauce	.10
catsup	.25	salad dressings		spaghetti sauce	.09
cheese sauce	.06	blue cheese	.07	steak sauce	.09
chili sauce	.24	caesar	.04	sweet & sour sauce	.45
hollandaise sauce	.08	French	.17	tartar sauce	.04
horseradish	.10	Italian	.07	tomato paste	.19
mayonnaise	.02	Russian	.07	Worcestershire sauce	.18
mustard	.04	thousand island	.15		

Sandwiches

BLT	.19	egg salad	.22	peanut butter & jelly	.50
chicken salad	.24	hot dog with bun	.26	tuna salad	.24
club	.13				

Fruits

apple	.13	fruit cocktail, in water	.10	persimmons	
applesauce	.10	grapes		Japanese	.20
appricots		concord	.14	native	.34
fresh	.13	European	.17	pineapple	
canned in water	.10	green, seedless	.14	fresh	.14
canned in juice	.14	grapefruit	.10	canned in water	.10
dried	.60	honeydew	.08	canned in juice	.15
banana	.20	lemons	.09	plums	
blackberries	.12	limes	.10	fresh	.18
cantaloupe	.08	mangoes	.17	canned in water	.12
cherries		nectarines	.17	prunes	
fresh, sweet red	.16	oranges	.12	dehydrated	.91
fresh, sour red	.14	papayas	.10	dried, cooked	.67
canned in water	.11	peaches		raisins	.77
maraschino	.29	fresh	.10	rasberries, fresh	.14
cranberry sauce, sugar	.36	canned in water	.08	strawberries	
dates, dried & pitted	.67	canned in juice	.12	fresh	.08
figs		pears		frozen, sweet	.26
fresh	.18	fresh	.15	tangerines	.12
dried	.62	canned in water	.09	watermelon	.06

Juices

apple cider	.14	grapefruit-orange		orange-apricot	.13
apple juice	.12	canned	.10	papaya	.12
apricot	.12	frozen	.11	pineapple	
apricot nectar	.15	lemon	.08	canned	.14
cranberry	.16	lemonade, frozen	.11	frozen	.13
grape		orange		prune	.19
bottled	.16	fresh	.11	tomato	.04
frozen	.13	canned, unsweet	.10	V-8	.04
grapefruit, fresh	.09	canned, sweet	.12		
canned	.07	frozen	.11		
frozen	.09				

Snack Foods

almonds	.19	marshmallows	.78	popcorn,	
cashews	.26	mixed nuts	.18	popped, no butter	.78
corn chips	.57	onion dip	.10	potato chips	.50
crackers		peanut butter	.17	pretzels	.75
graham	.73	peanuts	.20	sunflower seeds	
round	.67	pecans	.20	no shell	.19
rye	.50	pistachios	.19	walnuts	.15
saltines	.70				

Vegetables

artichoke	.10	carrots		peas	.12
asparagus	.04	raw	.10	peppers	.05
avacado	.05	cooked	.07	potatoes	
bamboo shoots	.05	cauliflower		baked	.21
beans		raw	.05	boiled	.15
raw green	.07	cooked	.04	hash browns	.29
cooked green	.05	celery	.04	French fries	.34
beans: kidney, lima,		chard, raw	.05	chips	.50
pinto, red, white	.21	corn		pumpkin	.08
bean sprouts	.06	steamed, off cob	.19	radishes	.04
beets, boiled	.07	sweet, creamed	.20	sauerkraut	.04
beet greens, cooked	.03	canned	.06	spinach	.04
broccoli	.06	cucumber	.03	soybeans	.11
brussel sprouts, cooked	.06	eggplant, cooked	.04	squash	
cabbage		lettuce	.03	summer, cooked	.03
raw	.05	mushrooms	.04	winter, baked	.15
cooked	.04	okra	.05	winter, boiled	.09
Chinese, raw	.03	onions	.07	tomatoes	.05
Chinese, cooked	.01	parsnips	.18	turnips	.05

Glycemic Index For Various Foods

**All foods are compared to glucose which was given a ranking of 100.
A faster rise in the blood sugar is seen with foods having a higher number.**

Breads		Fruit		Pasta Noodles	
pumpernickel	49	apple	38	macaroni	46
rye	64	banana	61	spaghetti, boiled 5"	33
white	72	orange	43	spaghetti, boiled 15"	44
whole wheat	72	orange juice	49	spaghetti, prot enrich	28
Beans		**Grains**		**Root Crops**	
baked beans	43	barley	22	potato, instant mash.	86
butter beans	33	brown rice	59	potato, mashed	72
chick peas	36	brown rice, instant	88	potato, new, boiled	58
frozen green peas	47	brown rice, parboil	44	potato, Russett	93
kidney beans	33	buckwheat	54	potato, sweet	50
red lentils	27	bulger	47	yam	54
dried soy beans	14	millet	75	**Snacks**	
Cereals		rye	34	corn chips	72
All Bran	54	sweet corn	58	oatmeal cookies	57
Cornflakes	83	wheat kernels	46	potato chips	56
Swiss Muesli	70	**Milk Products**		**Sugars**	
Oatmeal	53	ice cream	38	fructose	22
Puffed Rice	96	milk	34	honey	91
Shredded Wheat	70	yogurt	38	table sugar	64

Adapted in part from D.J.A. Jenkins, T.M.S. Wolever and A.L. Jenkins; Diabetes Care 11: 149-159, 1988

Index

With your physician's help, fill in the three tables below to set up starting basal rates and boluses, and a personalized sliding scale.

Use Table 7.1 To Fill In The Blanks Below And Find Your Starting Basal Rate And Boluses		
Your Weight	_____ lbs	
Basal Rate Estimated From Your Weight		_____ u/hr
Your Previous Average Total Daily Insulin Dose	_____ u/day	
Basal Rate Estimated From Your Previous Avg. Daily Insulin Dose		_____ u/hr
Lower Of The Two Estimated Basal Rates		_____ u/hr
Lower of The Two Carbohydrate Bolus Ratios		1 unit of Reg. for each _____ grams of CHO
Lower Of The Two High Blood Sugar Bolus Ratios		1 unit of Reg. for every _____ points over target

Table 7.2 Estimates For Starting Basal Rate And Boluses, Based On Weight And On Previous Total Daily Insulin Dose Using Injections

Starting Basal Rate(s)	
Time for Basal	**Basal Rate**
From 12 am to _____ __m	_____ u/hr
From _____ __m to _____ __m	_____ u/h
From _____ __m to _____ __m	_____ u/h
From _____ __m to _____ __m	_____ u/h
From _____ __m to _____ __m	_____ u/h
From _____ __m to _____ __m	_____ u/h
Comments: _____
_____
_____
_____

Blood Sugar	Sliding Scale Reg. Before Meals	Sliding Scale Reg. After Meals
< _____ mg/dl	No Extra	No Extra
_____ to _____ mg/dl	+ ___ unit	No Extra
_____ to _____ mg/dl	+ ___ unit	No Extra
_____ to _____ mg/dl	+ ___ unit	No Extra
_____ to _____ mg/dl	+ ___ unit	+ ___ unit
_____ to _____ mg/dl	+ ___ unit	+ ___ unit
_____ to _____ mg/dl	+ ___ unit	+ ___ unit
_____ to _____ mg/dl	+ ___ unit	+ ___ unit
_____ to _____ mg/dl	+ ___ unit	+ ___ unit
_____ to _____ mg/dl	+ ___ unit	+ ___ unit
_____ to _____ mg/dl	+ ___ unit	+ ___ unit
_____ to _____ mg/dl	+ ___ unit	+ ___ unit
_____ to _____ mg/dl	+ ___ unit	+ ___ unit
_____ to _____ mg/dl	+ ___ unit	+ ___ unit
_____ to _____ mg/dl	+ ___ unit	+ ___ unit
_____ to _____ mg/dl	+ ___ unit	+ ___ unit

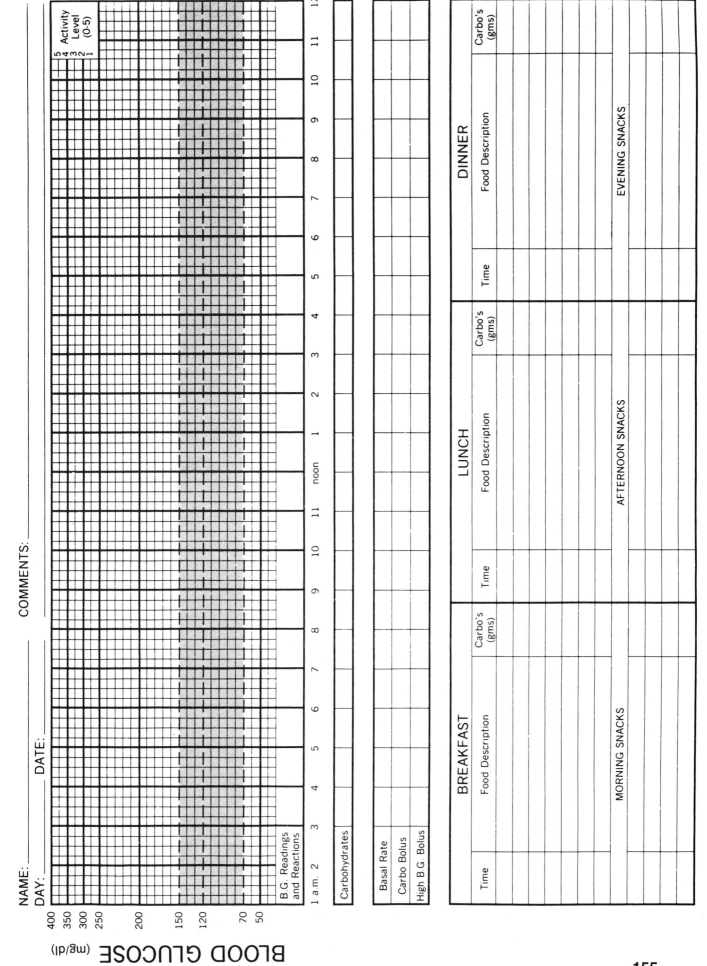

NAME: _____

DATE: _____

DAY: _____

COMMENTS: _____

BLOOD GLUCOSE (mg/dl)

	5
Activity	4
Level	3
(0-5)	2
	1

400
350
300
250
200
150
120
70
50

	1 a.m. 2	3	4	5	6	7	8	9	10	11	noon	1	2	3	4	5	6	7	8	9	10	11	12

B.G. Readings and Reactions

Carbohydrates

Basal Rate

Carbo Bolus

High B.G. Bolus

BREAKFAST

Time	Food Description	Carbo's (gms)

MORNING SNACKS

LUNCH

Time	Food Description	Carbo's (gms)

AFTERNOON SNACKS

DINNER

Time	Food Description	Carbo's (gms)

EVENING SNACKS

155

Order Form For *Pumping Insulin*

Please send me _____ copies of **Pumping Insulin** at $19.95 each. I understand that I may return any books for a full refund, for any reason. California residents add 7.0% sales tax ($1.40) for a total of $21.35. Discounts are available for 3 or more copies.

Name   _____

Address   _____

City   _____ State _____ Zip _____

Phone   (   ) _____--_____

        _____ copies of **Pumping Insulin** at $19.95 each (or $21.35 in Calif.)

Shipping: $2.50 for the first book, $1.00 for each additional book
Foreign surface mail: $5.00 for the first book, $3.00 for each additional book

Total $ _____   Payment: ❑ Check   ❑ Moneyorder

Mail your order to: **Torrey Pines Press**
1030 West Upas Street
San Diego, Ca. 92103-3821
Fax: (619) 497-0900